ALSO BY TIM S. GROVER

Jump Attack

RELENTLESS

FROM GOOD TO GREAT TO
UNSTOPPABLE

TIM S. GROVER

with Shari Lesser Wenk

SCRIBNER

New York   London   Toronto   Sydney   New Delhi

Certain identifying characteristics have been changed.

SCRIBNER
A Division of Simon & Schuster, Inc.
1230 Avenue of the Americas
New York, NY 10020

First Scribner hardcover edition April 2013

SCRIBNER and design are registered trademarks of The Gale Group, Inc.,
used under license by Simon & Schuster, Inc., the publisher of this work.

For information about special discounts for bulk purchases,
please contact Simon & Schuster Special Sales at 1-866-506-1949
or business@simonandschuster.com.

The Simon & Schuster Speakers Bureau can bring authors to your live event.
For more information or to book an event contact the Simon & Schuster
Speakers Bureau at 1-866-248-3049 or visit our website at
www.simonspeakers.com.

Manufactured in the United States of America

17   19   20   18

Library of Congress Control Number: 2012046789

ISBN 978-1-4767-1093-8
ISBN 978-1-4767-1421-9 (ebook)

To my parents,

Surjit and Rattan Grover,

whose love and support taught me

what it truly means to be relentless.

Everything I have, everything I am,

is because of them.

Contents

CONTENTS

RELENTLESS

DON'T THINK

I t was 10:00 p.m. when the black Suburban pulled up to the security gates of Attack Athletics, my training facility on the West Side of Chicago. Not unusual. Pro athletes would show up at all hours to the place where Michael Jordan, Kobe Bryant, and Dwyane Wade had permanent lockers, where countless superstars would work out or play ball or just hang out with other guys who got it.

On this particular night, though, only one guy is in the gym, and no one else knows he's there. Not his team, not the media, not his family. His teammates are in a hotel two thousand miles away; reporters are blowing up his phone with calls and texts.

And it's the middle of the NBA playoffs, with less than seventy-two hours until he has to be back on the court.

The night before, the whole world watched him limp off the floor in pain. Now everyone wants to know the story. Is he okay? Can he play? "I'm fine," he said at the postgame press conference. "He's fine," said the coach, who has no idea where his star is tonight. "We'll get him

1

some treatment and he'll be good to go," said the GM, who already knows the player won't go near the team's training staff.

Finally, when he's alone in the privacy of his room at the team's hotel, he makes one call, to the confidential number saved in the phones of countless athletes around the world.

"Need some help," he says.

"How soon can you get here?" I answer.

Getting to me without anyone knowing is the easy part when you're an elite athlete: call for a plane, grab your security guy, and go, confidentiality guaranteed. Typically, the hard part comes when you arrive, whether you're in need of emergency intervention or a long-term program or a psychological kick in the ass. Some guys arrive thinking they're going to fill out paperwork and stretch a little, and within the first hour they've sweated through three T-shirts and they're puking in a trash can.

But that night, the player and I knew the real issue wasn't physical; it's the end of the season, everyone has injuries. I'm not going to fix anything major in a few hours, and the team's training staff could have handled the usual aches and pains. Let's be honest: you don't secretly charter a plane and fly two thousand miles to get iced and taped. We can adapt around the limitation—here's how you adjust your shot, push off this way, land that way, do this before the game, do that at halftime, get something done to the shoes. Ignore the pain for now. You're going to be uncomfortable, get used to it. Lay out the whole script, leaving nothing to chance; if he follows the plan, he'll be physically ready to play. Or as ready as he can be.

But mentally, that's another story . . . and that's why he made the call to me. He's listening to all the talk about whether he'll be ready to go, whether he can get the job done, whether he's lost a few steps. And now he's not even sure himself.

The pressure is getting to him. External pressure that distracts and derails, not the internal pressure that can drive you to overcome anything.

And instead of shutting it all out and trusting his instincts and natural ability, he's thinking.

He flew two thousand miles to hear these two words: *Don't think.*

You already know what you have to do, and you know how to do it.

What's stopping you?

To be the best, whether in sports or business or any other aspect of life, it's never enough to just get to the top; you have to stay there, and then you have to climb higher, because there's always someone right behind you trying to catch up. Most people are willing to settle for "good enough." But if you want to be unstoppable, those words mean nothing to you. Being the best means engineering your life so you never stop until you get what you want, and then you keep going until you get what's next. And then you go for even more.

Relentless.

If that describes you, this book is your life story. You're what I call a Cleaner, the most intense and driven competitor imaginable. You refuse limitations. You quietly and forcefully do whatever it takes to get what you want. You understand the insatiable addiction to success; it defines your entire life.

If that doesn't describe you yet, congratulations: you are on a life-changing journey to discover the power you already possess.

This isn't about motivation. If you're reading this book, you're already motivated. Now you have to turn that into action and results.

You can read clever motivational slogans all day and still have no idea how to get where you want to be. Wanting something won't get you anywhere. Trying to be someone you're not won't get you anywhere. Waiting for someone or something to light your fire won't get you anywhere.

So how are you going to get there?

Believe this: Everything you need to be great is already inside you. All your ambitions and secrets, your darkest dreams . . . they're waiting for you to just let go.

What's stopping you?

Most people give up because everyone has told them what they can't do, and it's easier to stay safe in the comfort zone. So they sit on the fence, unable to decide, unable to act.

But if you don't make a choice, the choice will be made for you.

It's time to stop listening to what everyone else says about you, telling you what to do, how to act, how you should feel. Let them judge you by your results, and nothing else; it's none of their business how you get where you're going. If you're relentless, there is no halfway, no could or should or maybe. Don't tell me the glass is half-full or half-empty; you either have something in that glass or you don't.

Decide. Commit. Act. Succeed. Repeat.

Everything in this book is about raising your standard of excellence, going beyond what you already know and think, beyond what anyone has tried to teach you. Kobe says he wants six rings? I want him to have seven. A guy tells me he wants to come back from an injury in ten weeks? I'll get him there in eight. You want to drop thirty pounds? You'll drop thirty-four. That's how you become unstoppable—by placing no limits on yourself. Not just in sports, but in everything you do. I want you to want more and get everything you crave.

I don't care how good you think you are, or how great others think you are—you can improve, and you will. Being relentless means demanding more of yourself than anyone else could ever demand of you, knowing that every time you stop, you can still do more. You must do more.

The minute your mind thinks, "Done," your instincts say, "Next."

What you won't find in this book is a lot of garbage about "passion" and "inner drive." I don't have any feel-good strategies for dreamers who love to talk about "thinking outside the box." There is no box. I'm going to show you how to stop thinking about how you're going to think, and do something instead.

In these pages, you'll hear a lot about champions such as Michael Jordan and Kobe Bryant and Dwyane Wade, and many other successful people in and out of sports. But this isn't a basketball book, and I'm not going to tell you how to be the next Michael Jordan. No one will ever be Michael Jordan, and Kobe and Dwyane will be the first to agree. Will you ever play basketball like any of those guys? Probably not. Can you learn from their work ethic and relentless drive and uncompromising focus on their goals? Absolutely. Can you improve your chances of success by learning about others who succeeded, and those who didn't? Of course.

Success isn't the same as talent. The world is full of incredibly talented people who never succeed at anything. They show up, do what they do, and if it doesn't work out, they blame everyone else because they believe talent should be enough. It's not. If you want to be truly successful, you can't be content with "pretty good." You need to find an extra gear.

Look, I'm not a psychologist or a psychiatrist or a social worker. I didn't sit in a classroom for decades doing studies and collecting data to analyze and writing papers on the theories of excellence and elite performance. But I guarantee you that everything I know, everything in this book, comes from unlimited access to some of the most excellent and elite performers in the world; I understand how they think, how they learn, how they succeed and fail . . . what drives them to be relentless. It's not all pretty, but it's all true. Everything I've learned from them, everything I teach them, I'm sharing with you here. It's not science. It's raw animal instinct.

This book is about following those instincts, facing the truth, and getting rid of the excuses that stand between you and your goals, no matter how complex and unattainable they may seem, no matter how many people tell you it can't be done. It *can* be done.

Here's the key: I'm not going to tell you how to change. People don't change. I want you to trust who you already are, and get to that Zone where you can shut out all the noise, all the negativity and fear and distractions and lies, and achieve whatever you want, in whatever you do.

To get you there, I'm going to talk about some provocative topics, and you'll get no apologies from me if that makes you uncomfortable. Success is about dealing with reality, facing your demons and addictions, and not putting a smiley face on everything you do. If you need a pat on the back and a "Good job!" to get your ass off the couch, this is not the book for you. Because if you want to be unstoppable, you have to face who you really are and make it work for you, not against you. Truly relentless people—the Cleaners—are predators, with dark sides that refuse to be taught to be good. And whether you know it or not, you *do* have a dark side. Use it well and it can be your greatest gift.

If you're aiming to be the best at what you do, you can't worry about whether your actions will upset other people, or what they'll think of you. We're taking all the emotion out of this, and doing whatever it takes to get to where you want to be. Selfish? Probably. Egocentric? Definitely. If that's a problem for you, read the book and see if you feel differently afterward.

From this point, your strategy is to make everyone else get on your level; you're not going down to theirs. You're not competing with anyone else, ever again. They're going to have to compete with you. From now on, the end result is all that matters.

In the case of my late-night visitor, he had lost his connection to that end result. He was so distracted by his fear of losing that he couldn't focus on what he had to do to win, couldn't stem the wave of frustration and emotion that was drowning all his natural ability and confidence. His negativity on the court was evident; he was rolling his eyes at his teammates and coaches, grimacing as if he were dying out there. His teammates began to see that, and suddenly they were like troops marching into battle without their leader, completely shutting down. That's how great teams lose: the leader doesn't show up. It happens in business every day, when the boss shows his frustration in meetings or snaps at his employees. He's not confident, he's not cool, he's not on his game, and it comes out in little ways he might think no one else perceives. But you can be sure everyone picks up on it and panics.

How do you prevent that panic from turning into a total collapse? Sometimes you need to step away and get back to that calm, cool place where you're in total control. Could my player have called me to fly to wherever he was? Sure, that happens every season with different guys. They know if they need me, I'm there. But in this case, the player knew he needed space, and he was willing to risk the consequences if he got caught leaving the team. He knew it was on him to get back in the Zone, that deeply personal space where you can quiet your mind until you have no thoughts, it's just you and your instincts, focused and unemotional. Where you feel no external pressure, just the internal pressure to prove yourself, over and over, because you want it for yourself, not anyone else.

"Forget about losing," I tell him, looking for that "click" behind the eyes when you know the guy gets it. "Forget about trying, because if you're just trying, then losing is still an option. You want to be the best? Then you ignore the pain and the exhaustion and the pressure to please everyone else. You don't let your enemies take your balls, you don't let them set up shop in your head. When all hell breaks loose on the outside, you barely notice; you're calm on the inside because you're ready, prepared, and the best at what you do. You don't tell anyone how you're going to handle the situation, you just handle it. Everyone else is panicking and choking, and you say, 'No problem.' You step on the other guy's throat, and you finish the fight.

"And afterward you don't explain how you did it. They won't understand, and they don't have to. Just take a moment alone to recognize what you accomplished, and move on to the next challenge."

By now it's early morning; his plane is waiting to take him back. "Finish it," I say again. Click. He gets it. Time to go.

He turns to his security guy and says, "We've just been to Oz."

Relentless is about achieving the impossible. I know for a fact that anyone can do it. When I was still in high school, just a 5'11" basketball player in Chicago, I was watching a North Carolina game on television and saw Michael Jordan for the first time. He was a skinny freshman with moves I had never seen, completely instinctive and natural; he just knew what to do out there without even thinking about it. I didn't know anything about him, but I knew this kid was going to be a superstar.

Several years later, I had a master's degree in exercise science and was working as a trainer at a Chicago health club, and Michael was still skinny, but now he was a superstar with the Chicago Bulls. I had contacted the Bulls numerous times in the 1980s when I became a trainer, hoping for a shot at working with any of the players. I wrote letters to every player *except* Michael because I figured if he wanted a trainer, he would already have one, and it wouldn't be a guy like me who was just getting started. No one was interested. At that time, basketball players still weren't into weight training; the old-school belief was that a bulky upper body would mess up your shot.

Then in 1989, I saw a small newspaper story about how Michael was sick of being outmuscled by the world champion Detroit Pistons and the rest of the league. Once again I contacted the Bulls and talked my way into a meeting with the team doctor, John Hefferon, and the head athletic trainer, Mark Pfeil. What were the chances they would advise their superstar player to work with this unknown trainer who had never trained a professional athlete? None, everyone said. Forget it. Impossible.

Of course, everything is impossible until someone does it. Michael had worked with a trainer once, injured his back during the workout, and was hesitant about trying again. Yet he also instinctively knew it wasn't enough to have the greatest basketball skills in the history of the game. If he wanted to be more than a legend, if he was truly going to become an icon, he would also need to take his body to the ultimate level, and he was willing to do whatever was necessary to make that happen. So he told John and Mark to find someone who understood exactly what he needed.

A few days after my first meeting with the Bulls, they called me to meet again at their suburban practice facility. I figured it was another interview with the training staff. I had no idea I was being taken to a meeting with Michael Jordan at his home.

Michael and I talked for an hour, and I laid out the whole plan, showing him how we would slowly make him stronger and minimize the risk of injury, explaining how every physical change would affect his shot and how we would make adjustments along the way, getting his whole body working in balance for maximum peak performance, and probably extending his career.

He listened closely to everything I had to say before he responded.

Not possible, he finally said. It's too good. It just doesn't sound right.

It's right, I told him: "I'll give you a thirty-day schedule detailing exactly what we're going to do, how it's going to affect your body, your game, your overall strength. I'll tell you how you're going to feel so you can adjust to the changes we're going to make. We'll plan what you'll eat, when you'll eat it, when you'll sleep. We'll look at every detail, leaving nothing to chance. You'll see how everything works together."

He gave me thirty days.

I stayed for fifteen years.

When he finally retired, he said, "If I ever see you in my neighborhood again, I'm going to shoot you."

We learned from each other. We never saw obstacles or problems, we only saw situations in need of solutions. And since there had never been a player like Michael Jordan, we encountered a lot of situations without known solutions. We learned, we made mistakes, we learned from our mistakes. We kept learning.

Michael wasn't the best because he could fly through the air and make impossible shots; he was the best because he was relentless about winning, relentless in his belief that there's no such thing as "good enough." No matter how many times he won, no matter how great he became, he always wanted more, and he was always willing to do whatever it took—and then some—to get it.

For more than two decades, those values have been the cornerstone of all my work with hundreds of athletes, and now they are the cornerstone of this book. *Relentless* is about never being satisfied, always driving to be the best, and then getting even better. It's about finding the gear that gets you to the next level . . . even when the next level doesn't yet exist. It's about facing your fears, getting rid of the poisons that guarantee you will fail. Being feared and respected for your mental strength and toughness, not just your physical abilities.

Whatever's in your glass, empty it right now, and let me refill it from scratch. Forget what you thought, what you believed, whatever opinions you have . . . we start over right now. Empty glass. Those last few drops are the mental barriers that will prevent you from being better. We're going somewhere completely new.

The Cleaner
You Are, the Dirtier
You Get

The night the Miami Heat beat the Oklahoma City Thunder to win the 2012 NBA Championship, I wrote a message on a slip of paper before the game and put it in my pocket. It was for my longtime client and friend Dwyane Wade.

Dwyane had called me after Game Two of the Finals, asking if I would fly to Miami to see if I could get him and his damaged knee through the rest of the series. I was surprised; we have a long, successful relationship, but we hadn't worked together for the last two seasons, in part because he had chosen to stay in Miami to train near his teammate LeBron James. But we had stayed in touch, and like all my clients, past and present, he knew I would always be there if he needed me.

A different player might not have made that call. He could have relied on LeBron to carry the Heat to the title, he could have tried coping with the pain, hoping his knee would give him just a couple more games. That's what most players would have done. But when a championship is on the line and you're a Cleaner, you don't let others carry the load, and you don't just hope it all works out. You make every possible move to put yourself where you need to be.

So with the series tied 1–1, I flew to Miami. It was obvious Dwyane's knee would require surgery after the season; we couldn't slap a quick solution on that. I told him I'd do what I could to make him feel stronger and more explosive for the next few days.

I also told him that his one championship ring from 2006 wasn't going to be enough; he would need at least three to have a career that would be considered meaningful.

But what I really wanted to say to him was this: *When you're one of the greatest athletes in your sport, you don't announce you're "old" at the age of thirty and ready to pass the team along to the younger guys. If you think old, you become old. It wasn't that long ago you won the NBA scoring title after fighting back from simultaneous knee and shoulder surgeries, willing yourself through our grueling two-month rehab that would have taken anyone else three months. You did that. Do not tell me you can't do this.*

For those next few days, we worked on things he hadn't done in a long time, sometimes until 2:00 a.m., alone in the arena away from teammates and media and all the other distractions. For the first time in too long, it was all about him. The Heat took Game Three, and then Game Four, to lead the series 3–1. One more win, or the battleground would move back to Oklahoma City and the Thunder's home-court advantage. It was time to finish the fight, right now.

A lot of our work was physical; his body was coming alive in ways he hadn't experienced in a long time. But as with all serious competitors, the key component was mental.

He needed to find his way back to being the real Dwyane Wade, and not just one of the acclaimed "Big Three" of the Miami Heat. He had become so accustomed to sharing the stage with LeBron and Chris Bosh and the rest of the team that he had forgotten where he came from, how hard he had worked to be one of the very best.

I don't believe in long, windy pep talks or speeches; anything that requires a long explanation probably isn't the truth. And when I say something to one of my players, he knows he's getting the truth.

On the night of Game Five, when the Heat won the title, the note in my pocket read:

"In order to have what you really want, you must first be who you really are."

I wanted him to feel that time when it wasn't about smoke or lights or hype or keeping everyone else happy. When it was all about what happened on the court, when he fought with his life to get there, when anyone who fucked with him would get a forty-eight-minute blast of controlled rage. It was time to trust what he felt inside, not what everyone else was telling him to feel. *That's your name on the jersey. Remind them who you are. Go get what's yours.*

That night, as the young and determined OK City Thunder tried and failed to fight back from elimination, Dwyane was all killer instinct, deep in that Zone where he's explosive and dominant and aggressive. Others would have great performances—Mike Miller and Shane Battier and others raised their games beyond all expectations— but as the minutes ticked down, it was Dwyane's cool, intense confidence and commitment and leadership that earned the championship and got him that second ring.

I never gave him the note. I didn't have to.

That night, he was relentless.

Being relentless means never being satisfied. It means creating new goals every time you reach your personal best. If you're good, it means you don't stop until you're great. If you're great, it means you fight until you're unstoppable.

It means becoming a Cleaner.

We're all used to hearing about the Closer as the ultimate competitor, the guy you can always count on to finish out the game or make the deal or get you whatever you need. The Closer does what he's supposed to do, gets the credit, and goes home a happy hero.

Forget that. Think bigger. There's a level even higher, completely attainable but so special that most people don't even dare to dream of it.

Think Michael Jordan, the ultimate Cleaner.

Michael never cared about achieving mere greatness. He cared about being the best. Ever.

There's nothing wrong with being great. It's better than being good. Being great means you excel, which is hard to accomplish and something to be proud of.

But it doesn't make you the best.

Greatness makes you a legend; being the best makes you an icon. If you want to be great, deliver the unexpected. If you want to be the best, deliver a miracle.

This isn't just about sports performance; there are Cleaners in all walks of life. Look at the elite of any group—the top athletes or wealthiest CEOs or smartest students or strongest firemen, it doesn't matter—and it's fairly obvious that while they're all great at what they do, some will always perform on a different level. Look at the famed 1992 Dream Team, with eleven Hall of Famers; you can probably separate a couple from the rest. They all had talent. But a couple of them will forever be considered among the best of all time.

Michael set the standard for killer instinct and competitive drive. Each time his Chicago Bulls sealed another championship—there were six—he wouldn't just hold up the number of fingers for the rings he had already won; he'd hold up an extra finger for the next championship. After the first win he held up two, after the second he held up three . . . after the fifth he held up six. We'd be back in the locker room, champagne dripping down the walls, and he'd already be telling me what we needed to work on for the next season. A full year before he took his brief sabbatical to play baseball, he was already buzzing in my ear about baseball workouts. Never satisfied, never content, always pushing higher and higher.

That's a Cleaner.

Larry Bird is a Cleaner. Kobe, Dwyane . . . Cleaners. Pat Riley. Phil Jackson. Charles Barkley. There are a handful in the game today, not too many, and probably not whom you'd suspect—stardom doesn't automatically make you a Cleaner, winning does, and not just winning once; you have to be able to do it again and again. In the business world, we're talking about Bill Gates, the late Steve Jobs. Most team owners are Cleaners—guys such as Jerry Jones and Mark Cuban and Jerry Reinsdorf, who run their teams with the same cutthroat attitude that made them juggernauts in business. Most presidents are Cleaners, and good luck getting reelected if you're not.

There are others, in all walks of life; I'll let you consider the possibilities. Remember, it's not about talent or brains or wealth. It's about the relentless instinctive drive to do whatever it takes—anything—to get to the top of where you want to be, and to stay there. Dwyane wasn't the most gifted player on the floor the night the Heat won the title, but he was the only one who knew what everyone else had to do in order for them to win. That's what champions do; they put people in place to get results and make everyone else around them look better.

A Cleaner's attitude can be summed up in three words: *I own this.* He walks in with confidence and leaves with results. A Cleaner has the guts and the vision to steer everything to his advantage. You never know what he's going to do, but you know something's coming and all you can do is wait and watch, with fear and respect for his ability to handle anything without discussion or analysis. He just knows.

Being a Cleaner has almost nothing to do with talent. Everyone has some degree of talent; it doesn't always lead to success. Those who reach this level of excellence don't coast on their talent. They're completely focused on taking responsibility and taking charge, whether they're competing in sports or managing a family or running a business or driving a bus; they decide how to get the job done, and then they do whatever is necessary to make it happen. These are the most driven individuals you'll ever know, with an unmatched genius for what they do: they don't just perform a job, they reinvent it. *I own this.* I'm talking about the waiter who knows what every one of his customers drinks and how they order their steaks. Everyone in town wants to sit at his tables, and they all leave huge tips because they appreciate the excellence. I'm talking about the schoolteacher who won't give up until every student understands the lessons; the administrative assistant who earns more than some executives by knowing what the boss needs before the boss even realizes it; the parent working overtime to pay the bills and send the kids to college. It's the bus driver who gets on his bus every day, knows all the passengers, where they get on and where they get off, always smiling and friendly, but silently thinking, *This is my fucking bus and there will be no fucking around on my bus; it will be clean and on time, and anyone who messes with me or my bus will be back on the street walking.*

Navy SEALs are Cleaners. They lock in on their mission and stop at nothing to execute it; they know what has to be done, and it gets done. They expect to succeed, and when they do, they never celebrate for long because there's always more to do. Every accomplishment is just a stepping-stone to the next challenge; as soon as they've hit their target, they're already stalking their next conquest. Most of their work is done quietly behind the scenes, alone, without fanfare or glamour. Cleaners don't do it for show, they don't go through the motions. A true Cleaner never tells you what he's doing or what he's planning. You find out after the job is complete. And by the time you realize what he's accomplished, he's already moved on to the next challenge.

Why do I call them Cleaners? Because they take responsibility for everything. When something goes wrong, they don't blame others because they never really count on anyone else to get the job done in the first place. They just clean up the mess and move on. Think about the custodian who quietly works alone, late at night. He calls no attention to himself, no one sees him work, no one knows what he does, but the job always gets done. It has to, so everyone else can do their jobs efficiently. In his own way, he's the most powerful guy in the building: He has unlimited access, he knows where everything is and how it all works. He has the keys to every single door; he can go anywhere, unseen. He knows what everyone else is doing, all the dirty little secrets: who didn't go home, who snuck in late at night, who left the empty whiskey bottle under the desk, who left condom wrappers in the trash. If you have an emergency, he's the guy you call.

The Cleaner is never the first person you bring in; he's

the last, when it's finally obvious that no one else can handle the situation. No conversation, no panic, no discussion.

Cleaners are rule-breakers when they have to be; they only care about the end result. When things go wrong and everyone else starts to panic, the Cleaner is calm and unflappable, cool and steady, never too high or too low, never too happy or too depressed. He never sees problems, only situations to resolve, and when he finds the solution, he doesn't waste time explaining it. He just says, "I got this." And when it's over and he gets the results, all the others just stand there, shaking their heads in disbelief, wondering how he did it. Failure is never an option; even if it takes years, he'll find a way to turn a bad situation to his benefit, and he won't stop until he succeeds.

Cleaners have a dark side, and a zone you can't enter. They get what they want, but they pay for it in solitude. Excellence is lonely. They never stop working, physically or mentally, because it gives them too much time to think about what they've had to endure and sacrifice to get to the top. Most people are afraid to climb that high, because if they fail, the fall will kill them. Cleaners are willing to die trying. They don't worry about hitting the ceiling or the floor. There is no ceiling. There's no floor either.

Cleaners can't be invented by media or hype; they're self-made, and whatever they have, they've earned it. They're never in it for the money; the worst thing a Cleaner can do is sell out. He knows what he's worth, and he'll remind you if you make the mistake of forgetting. But the money is secondary to what really drives him, because here's the most important thing about a Cleaner, the one thing that defines and separates him from any other competitor: He's addicted to the exquisite rush of success. His lust for it is so powerful, the craving is so intense, that he'll alter his entire life to get it. And it's still never enough. As soon as he feels it, tastes it, holds it . . . the moment is over and he craves more.

Everything he does is to feed that addiction. It's not that he loves the process, he just loves that end result. I know you've absorbed a lifetime of advice about this: "Love what you do and you'll never work a day in your life!" Or "Love what you do and the money will follow." That might be true for some people, but not for a Cleaner. The idea of "loving" what he does would mean he was content, and a Cleaner is never, ever, content. Cleaners understand they don't have to love the work to be successful; they just have to be relentless about achieving it, and everything else in between is a diversion and a distraction from the ultimate prize. To an athlete, it means endless hours in the gym training and sweating and hurting. To a business owner, it's the time away from home and family, sacrificing a personal life for professional gain. For the teacher, it might mean untold unpaid hours getting every student through four years of high school and into college. The result is all that matters.

Eventually, though, all Cleaners have to walk away from their addiction before it completely consumes and destroys them. A Cleaner is all about control, and as soon as he feels the addiction is controlling him and not the other way around, he'll back off until he can regain control. That's why you see highly charged athletes, coaches, CEOs, and other extremely intense and driven individuals step away once they become the best of the best; the pressure to go even higher becomes too consuming. So they pull back, refocus, and usually return with a renewed appetite for even more.

But here's the good news, before you run away thinking you can't possibly live your life this way: It's not necessary—or even possible—to be a Cleaner in all aspects of your life. You don't have to be relentless about everything, you don't have to be the best at everything. You can't be unstoppable in your career *and* your relationships *and* your other interests, because achieving excellence in any one of those areas requires you to say, "I don't give a damn about anything else." If you're trying to be a Cleaner in business, you'll probably sacrifice your personal relationships. If you're a Cleaner in sports, you likely won't excel in business. If you want to be a Cleaner parent, your career will take a hit. Cleaners sacrifice the rest to get what they want the most. Most people stress about that. A Cleaner never does.

Cleaners don't care about "having it all." You ever see some of these billionaires? They're the worst-dressed guys in the room. Warren Buffett still lives in the house he bought in 1958 for $31,500. True Cleaners don't care about the bling and the showy lifestyle; they look at the bottom line. All that matters is the end result, not the instant gratification along the way.

• • •

In my work with elite athletes, I have to know whom I'm dealing with, their mental strengths and weaknesses, how far I can push them, how far they're willing to go. One day during the off-season I looked around my gym at a dozen All-Stars and another dozen potential All-Stars, all playing in our NBA-caliber summer pickup games. Every player there was considered "great," yet each performed at a different level with different motivations and limitations. Some were willing to go full strength every quarter, others were content to just play a little summer ball. And that's fine with me, but I pay close attention to the subtle differences that show me how serious someone is about getting ahead of everyone else. Let's face it: At the highest level of success in any area, everyone has reached some degree of outstanding achievement, so we're talking about shades of greatness. But if you want to be the very best of the best, it's the details that make the difference.

So just for my own thinking, I devised a three-tiered system that I've never shared with anyone prior to writing this book, categorizing different types of competitors:

Coolers, Closers, and Cleaners.

Good, Great, and Unstoppable.

You can apply these standards to any group of individuals; just look around your team, your office, your friends, your family. Everyone has a different definition of personal success: some people allow life's circumstances to decide for them, others decide what they want and say "good enough" when they get it, and then there are a select few who can't even define success because they keep raising the bar on what that means. Coolers, Closers, Cleaners. You'll consistently find that most people are Coolers, a smaller percentage are Closers, and maybe, just maybe, there's a Cleaner in the group. But if there is, you probably won't realize it until the first time you see him in action, and then you'll never forget.

A Cooler is careful; he waits to be told what to do, watches to see what everyone else is doing, and then follows the leader. He's a mediator, not a decision-maker; he's not taking sides unless he's forced to. He can handle a certain amount of pressure when things are going well, but when things get too intense, he kicks the problem over to someone else. He can make a huge play, but he's not ultimately responsible for the outcome. He's the setup guy, keeping things cool until the Closer or Cleaner can take over.

A Closer can handle a lot of pressure; he'll get the job done if you put him in the right situation and tell him exactly what you need him to do. He'll study all sorts of scenarios so he can anticipate what might happen, but he's uncomfortable when faced with something unexpected. He seeks attention and credit, and he's very aware of what everyone else is doing and what others think of him. He loves the rewards and perks associated with his fame and would choose financial security over winning or success.

A Cleaner is rarely understood, and he likes it that way.

Here's what I'm talking about:

- Coolers can have an amazing game.
- Closers can have an amazing season.
- Cleaners have amazing careers.

- Coolers worry about the competition and how they measure up.
- Closers study the competition and plan their attack based on the opponent.
- Cleaners make the competition study them; they don't care whom they're facing, they know they can handle anyone.

- Coolers avoid taking the winning shot.
- Closers take the shot if they know they have a good chance of making it.
- Cleaners just trust their gut and shoot; they don't have to think about it.

- Coolers won't offer to take on a role they're not comfortable with.
- Closers will take the role if you ask them and they'll do it well, if they have enough time to prepare for and study the situation.
- Cleaners don't wait to be asked, they just do it.

- Coolers let others decide whether they're successful; they do the job and wait to see if you approve.
- Closers feel successful when they get the job done.

- Cleaners never feel as if they've achieved success because there's always more to do.

- Coolers don't want to carry the team, but they're the first to slap you on the back when you do a good job.
- Closers want the credit for getting the job done and love being congratulated for what they did.
- Cleaners rarely congratulate you for doing your job, they just expect you to do it.

- Coolers think they want the spotlight, but when they get it, they usually handle it badly.
- Closers stand in front because they need to show who's in charge.
- Cleaners don't have to show who's in charge— everyone already knows.

- Coolers will eat whatever you feed them.
- Closers will order what they want and be satis-fied with a great meal.
- It doesn't matter what a Cleaner eats, he'll still be hungry again in an hour.

The Closer can win the game if given the opportunity, but the Cleaner creates the opportunity. The Closer can be the star, but the Cleaner maneuvered him into the job. Cleaners never need a kick in the ass. Everyone else does.

Good, Great, Unstoppable.

• • •

Are you a Cleaner?

Almost every Cleaner I've ever known—and I have known plenty—shares some combination of the traits below. You don't have to identify with all these things all the time, but I have no doubt you've experienced at least a few of them at some point. Some will intrigue you, some might repel you. But all of them will define your ability to be relentless.

There are thirteen, to remind you there's no such thing as luck. There are circumstances and outcomes, and you can control both if you desire. But if you insist on relying on luck, do it as the great Wilt Chamberlain did, believing his #13 wasn't unlucky for him, it was unlucky for his opponents. That's how a Cleaner thinks.

As you'll see, each is labeled #1, because if you give people a numbered list, they think #1 is the most important and the rest just follow behind. If it's a long list, they lose interest after #3 or #4. But on my lists, everything is equally important. If I give a player a list of things he must do to stay strong and healthy, and he skips any step, none of it works. So I don't number anything #1, #2, #3, #4 . . . I number everything #1.

The same is true for this book. You can wander through these chapters in almost any order, and I think you'll find the last is as important as the first.

THE RELENTLESS 13

When You're a Cleaner . . .

#1. You keep pushing yourself harder when everyone else has had enough.

#1. You get into the Zone, you shut out everything else, and control the uncontrollable.

#1. You know exactly who you are.

#1. You have a dark side that refuses to be taught to be good.

#1. You're not intimidated by pressure, you thrive on it.

#1. When everyone is hitting the "In Case of Emergency" button, they're all looking for you.

#1. You don't compete with anyone, you find your opponent's weakness and you attack.

#1. You make decisions, not suggestions; you know the answer while everyone else is still asking questions.

#1. You don't have to love the work, but you're addicted to the results.

#1. You'd rather be feared than liked.

#1. You trust very few people, and those you trust better never let you down.

#1. You don't recognize failure; you know there's more than one way to get what you want.

#1. You don't celebrate your achievements because you always want more.

If that list makes you nod and think, "So it's not just me," you're already on your way to being a Cleaner.

You'll see yourself in the chapters that follow, as we look more closely at each of the traits that form the platform of your success.

But I also know you might be thinking, Why? What's the upside? Never satisfied and driven by an addiction to success that never relents? Why put a value on being uncomfortable and alone? Why would anyone crave more pressure, more stress, more intensity?

I'll tell you why: because the reward is just so fucking good.

You do all of this to achieve what few others will ever comprehend or accomplish.

I won't ask you to transform into something you're not and don't aspire to be. I simply ask that you open your mind to the possibility that you can do so much more with what you already have. If you're serious about going where you've never been, pushing higher and further than you or anyone else thought you could, it's time to trust the voice inside telling you to do what you know you can do and become truly relentless.

#1. When You're
a Cleaner . . .

. . . You keep pushing yourself
harder when everyone else
has had enough.

_____

When you work with highly successful, high-profile people, there's a saying you live by or you won't be in that world for long: those who talk don't know, and those who know don't talk.

I don't talk.

My clients have enough exposure in their lives; they have to know that what we do in their private training belongs to them. If I don't have their complete trust, nothing gets done.

For that reason, little has ever been revealed about how I train my players, what goes on in the gym and everywhere else we work, and how we get the results that make the best even better.

But if you're willing to take this journey into the world of intense competition and achievement, I'm willing to talk about what I've learned from working with the greats for more than two decades, how I work with my athletes and how I've come to know what I know, what they've taught me and what I teach them.

I want you to be able to take all of this and use it as a framework for yourself to achieve whatever you desire. You don't have to worry about training like a professional athlete—that's a full-time job, and anyone who says you can "train like a pro" by reading a book is just trying to sell you a book. The book might be a good start, but let's be honest: you train like a pro by committing to work at the highest level of intensity, every moment, in everything you do, constantly working on your body, your skills, your preparation, leaving no detail to chance. It's not something you can do for thirty minutes in the morning, then head to work or school or wherever your other obligations take you.

But you can take an elite athlete's mentality and use it to succeed at whatever you do. Absolutely everything in this book can be applied equally to athletics or business or school or anything else you do in the world.

Because no matter what you want for yourself, whether your ambitions take you to the gym or the office or anywhere else you want to be, your ultimate power source will come from the neck up, not the neck down.

In sports, we spend so much time on the physical

component—training, working, pushing the human body to be faster and stronger and more resilient than most people ever thought possible. And then eventually, we get around to paying some peripheral attention to mental conditioning.

That's completely backward. Excellence isn't only about hitting the gym and working up a sweat; that's the smallest part of what you have to do. Physical ability can only take you so far.

The fact is, you can't train your body—or excel at anything—before you train your mind. You can't commit to excellence until your mind is ready to take you there. Teach the mind to train the body.

Physical dominance can make you great. Mental dominance is what ultimately makes you unstoppable.

You will never have a more powerful training tool than this: get your mind strong, so your body can follow. The true measure of an individual is determined by what you can't measure—the intangibles. Anyone can measure weight, height, physical strength, speed . . . but you can't measure commitment, persistence, or the instinctive power of the muscle in your chest, your heart. That's where your true works begins: understanding what you want to achieve and knowing what you're willing to endure to get it.

I want guys who want to work as hard as I do. I'm going to be relentless in my own pursuit of excellence, and I expect you to do the same. It's my name on the work we do together, and it's your name on the jersey. That better mean as much to you as it does to me.

And if you have to ask whether you can handle it, you can't.

When I train my athletes, it's a dictatorship with three rules: show up, work hard, and listen. If you can do those three things, I can help you. If you can't, we have no use for each other. I will bust my ass for you every way possible, but I expect you to do the same for yourself. I'm not going to work harder than you do for your benefit. Show me you want it, and I'll give it to you.

But we have to do this my way. No disrespect to your team trainer or dad or massage therapist, but if they knew how to handle the details of your situation, or if you knew how to do it yourself, you wouldn't be here. What we're going to do together is maybe 20 percent physical, and the rest is mental. You already have the talent; my job is to show you what you can do with all that talent so you can bust out of that cage holding you back. You may not like what I tell you, but if you stay with it, you'll see the rewards. Without a doubt, I've had plenty of players who aren't worth $2 million getting paid ten times that because they're in my program, they stick with it, and that means something to the teams. If you're working with me, they know you're serious.

If you're a professional, that means you're managing your career and we're going to approach it that way. Your body is a business you have to take care of, or the business goes away, and if you forget that, believe me, I will remind you. I'm not here to draft on your fame or your success. I expect us both to commit to hard work and dedication, and hopefully the result will be a professional relationship we can both be proud of. I see so many trainers who want to be friends with the players, trying to keep them happy for fear they'll lose a big-name client, going easy when the players say, "Enough." Believe me when I say this: I don't need to be your friend. You already have plenty of friends to tell you how great you are. What you and I do together is professional, not personal. If we end up being friends, that's great, but it's more important to me that we take care of your career and your future.

Some players like to be involved in planning what our work will entail; others are content to let me handle the details. Kobe wants to be part of figuring out what we have to do together; Michael was the same. Kobe will come to me and say something like, "Listen, when I jump off with my left leg I'm getting a pain in my knee." So I'll go back and retrace his steps: When did you start feeling it, what part of the game? Then I'll go to the video and replay everything he did, looking for something that might have affected that knee. Or was it something we did together working out? And I'll go through all the exercises to see if we might have aggravated something. I can say to him, "Remember in the Utah game, during this play, when this and that happened . . . ?" And he'll know what I'm talking about, we'll review the situation, until I can eventually say to him with some certainty, "I think your knee problem might have started there, and now we need to do this and that to fix it." Total collaboration.

So I'm happy to listen to your input and ideas, but once you're working with me, you agree to let me do what I do. No options. Most people have too many options, and they rarely choose the tougher one. Do you want to work out for ninety minutes or thirty minutes? Most people take the thirty minutes. Here, try this, but if it's too hard, we can make it easier. And they automatically make it easier. So I'm not giving you options. Nothing for you to think about. Let me do all the thinking for both of us. I'm making your life easy by doing all the homework and giving you the answers to the test. Just show up, work hard, and listen. That's your part of the deal. Do the work.

Do. The. Work. Every day, you have to do something you don't want to do. Every day. Challenge yourself to be uncomfortable, push past the apathy and laziness and fear. Otherwise, the next day you're going to have two things you don't want to do, then three and four and five, and pretty soon, you can't even get back to the first thing. And then all you can do is beat yourself up for the mess you've created, and now you've got a mental barrier to go along with the physical barriers.

For my guys, I'm the thing they don't want to do. For you, maybe it's something at the office or at home or at the gym. Either way, you have to do those things or you can't improve, you can't be the best, and you sure as hell can't call yourself relentless.

Cleaners do the hardest things first, just to show there's no task too big. They might not be happy about it, they don't ever love it, but they're always thinking about the destination, not the bumpy road that takes them there. They do whatever they have to because they know it's necessary, and you usually don't have to tell them twice.

More likely, while everyone else is slumped over in complete exhaustion, they'll want to do it all again, and then they'll say the second time was the best.

Of course, most highly successful people aren't accustomed to being told what to do. Yes, I know the team staff doesn't make you do this, that's the problem; they can't throw your ass out when you don't show up or you refuse to do the work. I can. The hot tubs, the cold tubs, the therapies, the late nights . . . once we're working together, it's not up to you. Cooperation is mandatory. If you big-time someone on my staff and refuse to get in that cold tub, he'll tell me so I can tell you, "Get in the fucking tub." And unless something dramatic has happened to you in the last twenty-four hours that I don't know about and you can change my mind, you're going to get in the tub.

Yes, I know it's uncomfortable. I'm not telling you to love it. I'm telling you to crave the result so intensely that the work is irrelevant. If it makes you feel better, I don't make things comfortable for myself either. I could take these great athletes, maintain their level of fitness, keep them healthy, and everyone would be content. But the challenge for me is taking someone great and making him even better. Michael, Kobe, Dwyane, my Hall of Famers—Hakeem Olajuwon, Charles Barkley, Scottie Pippen—and so many others . . . they come to me because they're not satisfied staying where they are, they're committed to enduring the pain and discomfort of improving on near-perfection, and they know I'll push them until they exceed their goals. If you start with someone average, someone with limited expectations, everything is an improvement. Anyone can do that job. But when you work with someone who's already the best in his field, the opportunity for improvement is a lot less obvious. I'm looking for every detail, every slight variable, to see what we can work on, anything to get the slightest edge. In the early days, I trained only Michael; later we added some Bulls teammates. Michael used to say, "I don't pay you to train me, I pay you not to train anyone else." He didn't want anyone else to get that edge.

And while that sounds flattering, here's the truth: no trainer or coach or expert can make you good or great or unstoppable if you're not going to do the work, if you're waiting for someone to make it happen for you. It's on you. And that's why I'm telling you all of this, not because I want you to know what I do for my guys, but because I want you to know what *you* have to do for yourself.

Bottom line if you want success of any kind: you have to be comfortable being uncomfortable. Every time you think you can't, you have to do it anyway. That last mile, the last set, the last five minutes on the clock. You have to play the last game of the season with the same intensity as you played the first. When your body is screaming and depleted and telling you, "No way, asshole," you work harder and tell yourself, "Do it. Now."

You control your body, it does not control you. You shut out the fear and emotion and physical stress and you do the thing you dread. You don't go through the motions and watch the clock until it's over. You invest in what you started, pushing yourself again and again beyond where you've already been.

This is not a Hollywood movie or a shoe commercial with a thumping sound track and special effects. No drama. No fantasy endings. If you want a feel-good story about a trainer bringing a guy from ruin to riches with a warm, fuzzy ending, go watch a *Rocky* movie. This is real life. If you pass out in the middle of one of my workouts, I'm not standing over you to coax you back onto your feet with compassion and support. I'm going to make sure you're breathing, and then I'm leaving you right there. When you finally come around and you've cleaned up your puke, come find me and we can get back to work.

We always get back to work.

I'm always thinking up new ways to see how I can push someone, shock the body and rock the mental stamina. If you do what you always do, over and over, you're always going to get the same result. My goal is to make it so challenging in the gym that everything that happens outside the gym seems easy. The work is about testing yourself and preparing all your options, so when you're performing, there's nothing to think about. Do the work before you need it, so you know what you're capable of doing when everyone else hits that panic button and looks at you. Anything you do with me will be so much harder than you'll ever experience in a game situation, you won't have to think about what's happening. You'll just know, and your body will follow.

You tell me your limit, and I'll show you how much more you can do. The question is, what *is* that limit? When Kobe suffered a broken nose and a concussion in the All-Star Game, he was insistent on playing in the Lakers' next game. Why? He had to know how his body would respond to the trauma, and what he was capable of doing under those circumstances. Few people know what they're truly able to accomplish, and even fewer want to find out.

Can I push you beyond your limit and not break you? How far can you go, and are you willing to go there? You have to be with me 100 percent, not thinking about what you're doing tonight or the bills you have to pay. Complete focus for complete results.

When I get focused with a client, I'm watching everything: facial expressions, heart rate, how he's sweating, which leg is shaking, everything down to the smallest detail. Then I take all that information, process everything, and decide: Am I willing to push this a little bit further? Because if I do, his progress is going to double in half the time. But he has to be willing to deal with what I'm asking of him.

A lot of my work has involved bringing athletes back from serious injuries and surgeries, and I always tell a player that when I return him to the game, he won't be the same as he was, he'll be better. He has to be better. Because if he comes back just as he was when he got hurt, he's probably going to get hurt again. So I make him do more than he's ever done and push him harder than he's ever worked, so he can be stronger and more powerful than he was before.

But that fear component is a powerful obstacle, and often when we first get started, these guys are just scared to move. For the first time in their lives, they can't rely on their physical abilities or control their own motion, and now they're afraid of their own bodies. It's one of the biggest obstacles to recovery; they no longer want to move. And when you're an athlete who doesn't want to move, you lose your hunger and focus, especially when there's a guaranteed contract with your name on it. Remember when you were a kid and an injury might have meant losing your spot on the team, so you fought like hell to come back to action? You'd throw some dirt on it and get back in the game. Not the case at the pro level. But only the individual knows whether he's ready. I don't care what an X-ray or MRI says; if he's not mentally ready, he's not ready.

So we go back to the fundamentals. We're going to walk, we're going to move your shoulder, we're going to take everything one step at a time. Small moves to rebuild your confidence. The small moves eventually add up to big changes. Every two or three days, we're going a little farther out on the limb, trying a little more, making progress.

But I'm not going to make it comfortable. Why should I? Comfortable makes you good. We're going for unstoppable, and there's a price to pay for that. I'm not going to hurt you, but if you don't trust me to take you where you have to go, we can't get this done. I'm never going to put you in a situation you're not ready for, but I'm going to put you in that situation quicker than most people would. Because if I allow you to get there at your own pace, we're never going to get there.

People are always asking me about the secrets and tricks I use to get results. Sorry if this disappoints you:

There are no secrets. There are no tricks. If anything, it's the opposite: Whether you're a pro athlete or a guy running a business or driving a truck or going to school, it's simple. Ask yourself where you are now, and where you want to be instead. Ask yourself what you're willing to do to get there. Then make a plan to get there. Act on it.

There are no shortcuts. I don't want to hear about workouts you can do in five minutes a day, or twenty minutes a week; that's total bullshit. Those workouts "work" for people who have never moved off the couch, and now they're moving for five minutes so they're burning a few calories here and there. Look, if you're three hundred pounds and you've never done anything, and I get you working out twice a week for a month, maybe you'll drop a dozen pounds. If you usually consume two bags of chips and a liter of soda every night, and then you drop down to only one bag of chips and a can of soda every night, your body might respond to the calorie reduction and drop a little weight. But I wouldn't call that "fitness," and I detest the so-called programs that lie to people and offer ridiculous promises based on nonsense. Don't tell me about a workout that's "easy" and done in the "comfort of your home." Any workouts involving the words *easy* and *comfort* aren't workouts. They're insults. You can work out at home, but if whatever you're doing makes you feel "comfort," something is very wrong.

This is your life. How can you not invest in that? I'm not just talking to the athletes here, but to anyone who places value on success. Picture a highly successful guy who has accomplished so much, but he's a hundred pounds overweight because he's driven by a food addiction he can't control, and he's content being an unhealthy multimillionaire. He's got all the financial success in the world, people admire and respect him for it, and he has no problem finding so-called friends to help him spend his money. But he's too fat to have decent sex or do other physical activity, he's going to drop dead twenty years early, and all his hard work will end up as someone else's inheritance. How's that financial success working then?

People refuse to work out or control their diets because it's not comfortable for them. But how comfortable can it be to drag around all that extra weight and all the physical problems that go along with it? Back pain, joint issues, shortness of breath, diabetes, heart problems . . . I'd estimate 85 percent of all physical discomfort comes from being overweight. Explain to me: If you can choose between being uncomfortable because you're overweight and sick, or uncomfortable because you're sweating at the gym three times a week, why do so many people choose the discomfort that leads to complete physical failure?

I get a lot of calls from guys who need to manage their weight. They've seen every nutritionist and dietician on earth, and they're still walking in with bags of fast food. But if you let me do what I have to do, we can get that weight off in a few weeks. We took a hundred pounds off Eddy Curry so he could sign with the Miami Heat in 2012, and we can help you with those thirty pounds you need to lose before training camp.

But you have to be willing to do the work. Last year I

got a call from a baseball agent whose client was a pitcher needing to drop forty pounds before spring training. One day before he was supposed to start the program I set up for him, he decided he'd rather take the weight off on his own. I asked him, Are you sure? It's not that easy to drop forty pounds, especially when you put the weight on over a lot of years due to bad eating and poor workout habits. No, he was sure, that was his decision. Good luck, I told the agent, he'll be out of the game in eight months.

I was wrong on that one, he was gone in four.

If you come to me to drop weight, you better have your last meal before we get started. I've got five weeks to get you in shape; we're starting the minute you walk in the door, and if you don't cheat, if you don't swipe a few fries off your buddy's plate or sneak a few beers at your cousin's wedding, you'll drop twenty pounds in the first three weeks. I'll give you the meals, I'll give you a list of everything you can eat and everything you can't. I'll send someone to cook for you. I'll sit down with your wife or mom and explain how much sugar is in the two gallons of orange juice you're putting down every day. But you have to follow the rules.

Believe me, if you really want to know what someone is made of, watch them go through sugar detox. This isn't a "low carb" diet or Atkins knockoff; we're talking zero sugars. And since most people have no idea how much sugar is hiding in most foods, I give them a written guideline of what they can and can't eat, with a warning that says, *You'll know the program is working when you get a headache right behind one eye and you want to throw up*. Within the first two days, they twitch, get hot and cold sweats, terrible gas, crazy thirst, and then they get shakes that only heroin and cocaine addicts can understand. I'm taking every ounce of sugar out of your body for ten days. After two horrible days, it starts getting better. And if you cheat, I'll know. I make all my trainers go through it so they know what it feels like.

A guy will come into the gym during his detox and I'll ask how he feels. Fine, he says, just fine. Hmm.

Next day I ask him again: How ya feeling? Feeling great, no problem, he says.

I give it one more day. Feeling okay? Following the diet? Yep, all good.

Okay, you're a fucking liar. You want to screw this up, do it somewhere else. I know it's not easy, but you can't stay in your comfort zone and expect results. Challenge yourself. Don't be afraid to be uncomfortable. We can't help people committed to failure.

I love the guys who want results so much they'll fight me to do more than they're supposed to. I'll tell them if they're not ready, but I'd rather see a guy trying to sneak in some extra work than blow off a workout because he has to go shoot a magazine cover or promote a shoe. The work they do with me makes all the other stuff possible. Not the other way around.

After Dwyane's knee surgery in 2007, he was in the weight room working on a drill that I make every player do after rehabbing from ankle, knee, or hip surgery before he gets the green light to play: stand on a forty-eight-inch padded cylinder, then jump down to the floor and up onto another forty-eight-inch cylinder. Not easy, physically or mentally. It shows me whether his body can withstand the stress, but equally important, whether his head is ready to trust his body, or if he's fearful about his ability to perform. Because the key isn't the physical challenge of jumping up, it's overcoming the fear of jumping down.

So Dwyane was going through this drill, with numerous other players working out nearby. A few days later, my trainers started telling me all the other guys were secretly trying it too, sneaking into the weight room when no one was in there, bounding up and down these cylinders just to see if they could do what Dwyane did. And most of these guys hated jumping drills, but they had to know how they measured up. With Cleaners, there's no off-switch. They're always on.

One of my biggest challenges is keeping the ball away from a guy who isn't supposed to be playing yet. When I get these great players recovering from injuries or surgeries, I set up a detailed plan for their rehab and return, and the *last* thing they're going to be allowed to do is walk onto the court. But try telling that to a guy who has never spent five minutes without a ball in his hand.

Perfect example: the great Charles Barkley, probably the most athletically gifted individual I've ever seen, and a Cleaner in every way. Charles was working with me after knee surgery, and he was not happy when I said he and his postsurgical torn patella had to stay off the court as long as he was in an immobilizer.

He looked at me with that death stare and demanded

a ball. Then he stood under the basket and dunked ten times off the healthy foot. Dunked. Ten times. One foot. The boot never touched the ground.

Those are the guys I want, the badasses who will take chances and push themselves. I can tell everything about a guy within the first three days of working with him. On the first day, he'll show up ready to go, and I'll make him work like he never worked before. The second day, when he wakes up feeling aches in body parts he didn't even know he had, it's going to be tempting to blow off our workout. But it's only day two and he's only sore in his upper body because that's what we worked on, so he'll usually show up for more. But by day three, after we've worked both the upper and the lower body and his muscles are screaming from the lactic acid, I'll know everything I need to know, because he's going to be completely miserable from the first two days. Forty-eight hours, that's the test. If he keeps showing up despite the pain and exhaustion, we're good to go. If he tells me he can't make it . . . he's in the wrong place. There are plenty of trainers out there who will work that way. Not me. Get comfortable being uncomfortable, or find another place to fail.

#1. When You're a Cleaner . . .

. . . You get into the Zone, shut out everything else, and control the uncontrollable.

A Cooler gets everyone cranked up and emotional before the game.
A Closer gets himself cranked up and emotional before the game.
A Cleaner never gets cranked up or emotional; he stays cool and calm and saves it all for game time.

Quiet, dark, alone. Always alone, even in a crowd, even when you're surrounded by an entire arena of fans screaming your name. Alone in your head, alone with that buzz no one but you can feel . . . no outside static. No distraction. Right now, all about you. That dark side pushing you, burning in you, driving you . . . do it. Do it. You can hear your heart, you control every beat. You control everything. Somebody is talking at you . . . but you don't hear and don't want to. Later tonight someone—media, colleague, family—will say you're a jerk, rude and uncommunicative. They don't get it and you don't care. "In your own little world," they say. Yes. Exactly. Get out. Leave me alone. Leave me alone.

You're in the Zone.

You know others around you are emotional. They feel scared or jealous or excited or they're too clueless to understand what's happening, but you feel only readiness. No emotion, because in the Zone the only sensation is anger, a quiet, icy anger simmering under your skin . . . never rage, never out of control. Silent, like a storm that moves in slow and dark, its violence unseen until it hits, and can't be measured until it moves on.

That's the impact of a Cleaner in the Zone.

Everything you feel, all your energy, it's right under the surface. No ripples, no waves . . . no one can see what's coming. Leave the drama and chaos to others, that's not you. You're saving it all for what's ahead.

Because once you step into the Zone, that's it. You own time.

For all the time we spend working on our careers and talents—going to school, building a business, making money, training the body—it's ultimately your mental focus and concentration, your ability to control your environment and the heartbeats of others, that determines whether you succeed or fail.

Think about this: In your two feet, you have 52 bones, 38 muscles and tendons, 66 joints, and 214 ligaments. And at the other end of your body, one lightweight brain, floating around in your head. You can find out almost everything about the intricate function of your bones, joints, ligaments, muscles, and tendons, and how they allow you to do what you do. But you can find out almost nothing about the intricate function of your brain, and *why* it allows you to do what you do.

Anyone who has experienced the awesome power of the Zone will tell you it's deeply calm. It's not relaxing or peaceful—this isn't yoga—but intensely focused. And once you're there, you have no fear, no worry, no emotion. You do what you came to do, and nothing can touch you. But what takes you to that elusive space where you're fearless and powerful, where you can completely trust yourself to just let go? How do you find that perfect internal silence that people talk about but can't ever really describe?

One thing I know for sure is that we all have a trigger that puts us in the Zone, something that ignites our competitive intensity, laser focus, and a relentless craving to attack and conquer. It's different in every individual, and no one can tell you how to get there. But I can tell you this much: it comes straight from the part of you I call your dark side, which we're going to discuss in the pages ahead. Truth: when you're finally able to let go and be who you really are, that's what puts you in the Zone, and only then can you control your fear and inhibition. Without that deep instinctive component, it's like trying to light a lighter that has no fuel inside. You get a lot of sputtering little sparks but no fire.

Part of what I do is help find the fuel to light that fire. I know it's there, and I know which buttons will set off the explosion. But I don't want to be the one who pushes those buttons; I want *you* to push those buttons for yourself, so you know how to set off the explosion on your own. So I'll go the other way: I pull those buttons way out and show you where they are so you can push them yourself when you're ready. I don't want you giving me or anyone else that kind of control; as soon as you allow others to push your buttons, they've won. The Zone belongs to you alone, and only you can decide how and when that fire gets lit.

But one way or another, we're gonna get it lit. Maybe I'll mention what another player did . . . and pull out that button for you. I'll repeat something I heard from the coach . . . another button ready to go. After an unbelievable performance, I'll ask what you did last night, because you need to do that again before the next game. Or I'll tell you I'm going back to the hotel to pack your bags because you're playing as if you've already left town. More buttons. Then I'll have someone get aggressive with you during a workout . . . and *boom*. That was the button you hit, and for the next hour, you can't be stopped.

Now you're in the Zone, and you may never recall how you got there and what happened once you arrived. For some, it's having their manhood or ability questioned. For others, it's the sight of their own blood. For some guys, it's a physical confrontation. I just keep pulling buttons until you have an arsenal to work with, and then I wait to see which one you punch to kick yourself into hyperspace. And once you show me what lights you up, I'm going to make sure you stay lit.

It's rare to actually see someone shift into the Zone; it usually happens privately and silently. But on rare occasions, that moment is suddenly on display as the world watches. During the 2012 Olympics, as Team USA played Australia, Kobe was having a surprisingly weak first half. It happens; a player has something else on his mind, just feels off, can't get focused for whatever reason. Most guys who start a game that way finish even worse. But the greats can recognize they need to turn it around, and that's what Kobe did, hitting four 3-pointers in just over a minute, leading the Americans to a 119–86 victory. "Just searching for something to activate the Black Mamba," he said after the game. Just finding his way back into the Zone.

Michael was the only player I've ever known who was completely in the Zone every time he played, always a Cleaner. Even in games where he'd cruise a little, it would eventually come out. I recall one night in Vancouver, during the Bulls' 72-win season, everyone was tired from the long annual November road trip, and it was a rare game when the Bulls were getting killed. By the fourth quarter Michael had only 10 points, and the Grizzlies' Darrick Martin started talking a little trash at him.

You never, ever, challenge Michael Jordan and expect to come out ahead. Michael literally stopped on the court.

Looked at the guy. Shook his head and said, "Let a sleeping dog lie." The dark side said, "Kill this motherfucker," and he went into attack mode, straight into the Zone. Result: unstoppable. He went on an unbelievable tear, scoring 19 points in the quarter on the way to a Bulls' win, and Darrick Martin spent the rest of the game on the bench.

Michael never cracked, never showed emotion. On occasion he'd show a positive expression, such as that infamous little "I can't help it" shrug after hitting six 3-pointers in a half against Portland in the playoffs, or the legendary hand-in-the-air moment against Utah. Always positive and upbeat, raising up the team and the fans and everyone else, showing he had everything under control. If he ever felt anything negative, he never showed it. That's a Cleaner.

If you're in the military and you see your commander backing up or if you're in an office and you see the boss becoming unhinged, what does that say to everyone else? Cleaners show emotion if it's the only way to get everyone else where they need to be. But never because the Cleaner has lost control of his feelings.

Before a game, I don't want to see guys dancing and shaking and screaming each other into a frenzy. It looks good for the fans and the cameras, but all that emotion pulls your focus toward manufactured pregame hype and away from your mission. And what happens right after that moment of insanity? It's over. Back to the sideline. Commercial break. Total letdown. Out of Zone.

Watch the true leaders. At game time, Kobe comes onto the court the way a CEO walks into a shareholders' meeting. Shakes a few hands, says hello to the players and the refs, and gets down to business. Michael wanted no physical contact before a game—no hugs or handshakes. He'd give his teammates a fist bump or a subtle high five—hands never too high, always low and contained—and he never made eye contact. At the end of the player introductions, he'd go around to his teammates and settle everyone down, like a father covering the kids, a quick moment to remind them, Don't worry, I got you.

A Cleaner is never going to stand up in front waving a towel; he's down at the end, alone, focused and unemotional. At a critical moment when everyone gets too pumped up and overheated, he's the guy telling everyone else to keep it cool.

No matter what was happening during a game, Michael always looked as if he were having the time of his life out there. When he stepped between those lines, nothing could touch him, nothing bothered him . . . that was his Zone. Most guys, everything touches them; when things go bad, they look as if they're dying out there. Michael stayed in the Zone 100 percent of the time, from the moment he left his home or hotel room for the game until the moment he returned late that night. But during that time on the court he was the real and authentic Michael. After the game, before he'd do an interview, he'd go into the trainer's room, where no reporters were allowed, get fully dressed, and switch from the authentic Michael who'd just played the game to the MJ everyone else perceived him to be.

Most people can't do that, nor do they want to; at

some point, it wipes you out to stay so intense and constantly charged, always a loner, always in a place no one can go but you. Eventually, you end up having to exhale, relax, let down that wall of intensity, fall out of the Zone. But once you're out of it, it's hard to get back in.

When you see someone lose connection with the Zone, it's as if the lights went out. Suddenly you see this guy go from a silverback to a pussycat because he's lost his confidence and forgotten who he is. That's how it was with Gilbert Arenas, whom I worked with after one of his knee surgeries. Just a great guy. When he was on top of his game, he was a total killer: you could tell him to go get you 25 points, turn him loose, let him do his thing, and he'd deliver. Not complicated, just let him go on instinct. He'd taunt you, step on you, completely destroy you. Almost like the old MJ days, where he'd just torture you into submission. But eventually I could see Gilbert slipping away; his personality on the court changed, as if he'd forgotten how to step on someone's throat. The people around him didn't know how to manage that, and he just declined.

It happens more than you think, a great player losing that ability to turn the key and tap those killer instincts. But usually it's because something has rocked the dark side of his life, and when it becomes public—such as becoming entangled in a scandal—it's painfully obvious why he's lost his focus. And the only way for him to get it back is if (a) something major and catastrophic happens to jolt him back there, or (b) he's so unapologetic about what happened that he doesn't care what anyone thinks or how it looks. Now he's the walking dead with nothing to lose, which makes him one of the most dangerous predators imaginable.

You can tell someone all day, "You need to relax, you need to focus." But what does that actually mean? You're not giving him anything he can use. He's looking for someone to tell him what he's doing wrong because he thinks he's relaxing and clearly he's not. I can always tell when something on the inside is making someone react on the outside. So I point it out. Here's your movement pattern, you look nervous. Your eye contact shows stress, you're looking away instead of looking at your opponent. You're grabbing at your shorts, you're rolling your eyes . . . you're emotional. And you're doubting yourself, so the other guys have done their job and set up shop in your head; they've pulled you off your game. You're not in the Zone.

You're thinking. Don't think.

When you're a Cleaner in the Zone, you operate with no wasted motion, no chaos, no warning. You don't tell anyone what's about to happen, it just happens. You may not even remember how it happened, but you know it did; as Kobe says, you know you're in the Zone but you can't think about it, because thinking is a distraction. Every movement has a purpose, and you know exactly what that purpose is; you're never killing time or going through the motions. You can look around you in any situation and see those who get it and those who don't. On a team, in business, in any group, you'll have those who are there for the paycheck, and those who understand the mission. As in an intricate military operation, everything has a reason and a result. A Cleaner operates out of pure desire for that result because he knows he must execute or fail. There is no other way.

Players always ask me what they should think about at the free throw line, something to make them forget the pressure, block out the crowd and the noise and all the distractions. First of all, I can't give you a made-up thought, it has to be something internal that means something to you. But ideally, I want you thinking about nothing. If you're truly in the Zone, it's just you and the ball and the hoop, as if you're alone on the playground or the driveway or the practice floor. I'd rather have you tell yourself, "It's just a couple of free throws, not the end of the world either way." But if you have to go somewhere in your head, go somewhere positive, to your kids or something that's all about pure relaxation and happiness.

You can control your own space, reconnect with your instincts, and refocus your energy in a lot of ways. If I'm trying to get you there, sometimes I'll try old music that brings back childhood memories or feelings, songs you may not have heard for ten years, but they take you to another place, when you felt a certain way that worked for you. I don't use the new stuff that gets you hyped up. I want you cool and relaxed, just being who you are, who you used to be before everyone started pressuring you to be different. There's an incredible physical response that's not about the music. It's just an instinct. There's a calming chill, and the heart rate drops from the resting rate to the rate when you're in the Zone, maybe two to three beats a minute slower, almost immediately. I'll know it's the right song when you smile . . . when we get it right, there's always a smile.

I'll keep at it until I know you're back on track, and then you have to take over from there. I don't want you relying on me or anyone else; I just want to point you in the right direction and then get the hell out of the way. Sometimes I'll give a guy a note, maybe while he's stretching or warming up, as I did with Dwyane in Miami, just to quiet his mind. Some guys arrange to see their kids at halftime or at the end of the game, a quick hug and kiss, something to relieve all the pressure, because the kids don't care if you score 2 points or 100 points, they just want the hug and kiss from Daddy. And for Daddy, it transfers some of the tension and emotion from the game into something calmer.

But once a Cleaner steps into the Zone, he's detached from everything on the outside. Whatever else is going on—personal, business, anything—it can't affect him until he's ready to return. That, by definition, is the Zone. No fear, no intrusion. Total concentration. You're not thinking, because thinking turns your thoughts *on* to everything, and the Zone is about the opposite, turning your thoughts *off* to everything except the task at hand. Thinking takes you away; the Zone keeps you where you need to be. That's your safe haven: you go inside that space, and nothing can touch you, nothing can hurt you, no one can call you or text you or hassle you or bother you. The headaches will still be there when you're done, but you have to get to that place where you control time and space, and nothing controls you.

If one thing separated Michael from every other player, it was his stunning ability to block out everything and everyone else. Nothing got to him; he was ice. No matter what else was going on—the crowds, the media, the death of his father—when he stepped onto that basketball court, he was able to shut out everything except his mission to attack and conquer. I've never seen another player form such a perfect boundary around himself, where nothing goes in except what he brings with him. Dwyane is probably the closest, when he's healthy; he's got that switch that allows him to step inside those lines and forget everything else. Most people though, even the greats, take some external stuff with them; few can leave it all behind.

When you consider that Michael's career shooting percentage was 50 percent—meaning the ball found its mark one out of every two times, with three guys hanging on him and twenty thousand cameras flashing every time he took a shot—you can begin to appreciate how deep in the Zone he was for every single game, every quarter, every play. There was no difference between what he did in practice and what he did in the game, his mechanics were consistent in any environment. I can't stand hearing athletes say, "When I'm under the lights, that's where I turn it on." No. When you're in the Zone, you shouldn't even notice the lights. Or need them.

But few people can duplicate that extreme level of focus and concentration in different settings; they become comfortable in one place, and that's where they perform the best. Why do teams play better at home than on the road? Why do some athletes perform better in certain stadiums than others? They can't reproduce that environment that puts them in the Zone. They're thinking about being in a different atmosphere, instead of instinctively knowing how to adapt to their surroundings. Instead of dictating the outcome of the event, they're letting the event dictate the outcome to them. Instead of feeling steady and steely, they start feeling unsure and worried. They lose their cool confidence, they start feeling emotional, and make no mistake about this: emotions make you weak.

Again: emotions make you weak.

The fastest way to tumble out of the Zone is to allow emotions to drive your actions.

When you feel fear, you recoil and put up a wall to protect yourself. Is there really a wall there? No, but you act as if there were. Now you can't go forward because of the wall. Put your hand through it, there's nothing there, you can walk straight through it. But if you stay behind that imaginary wall, you fail.

When you feel rage, you lash out. When you lash out, you're usually irrational because you're acting out of impulse, not reason. Now you're out of control and you've lost all sense of what you're supposed to be doing. Instead of feeling cool and prepared, you've lost all sense of focus. And without focus, you fail.

When you feel jealousy, you shift all your attention and energy to whoever is making you jealous. Doesn't matter if it's a colleague's success or your girlfriend's new man; either way, you're thinking about something other than what you're supposed to be doing. And you fail.

The only exception to the emotions rule is anger: controlled anger is a deadly weapon, in the right hands. I'm not talking about a raging volcano that can't be managed from inside or outside, but anger you can restrain and turn into energy. All Cleaners have that slow-burning, blue-hot internal anger, and it works if they can control and maintain it. But it never becomes blind rage, and it's never allowed to become destructive. When you channel anger the right way, you get Michael shaking his head in Vancouver and annihilating the game. He didn't slug anyone, he stayed steady and unemotional and turned his quiet anger into results.

But it's a fine line. If you don't control your anger, you get violent, throw a punch, argue with the refs, glare at the other players, get completely emotional, and stumble permanently out of the Zone.

Emotions pull your focus and reveal that you've lost control, and ultimately they destroy your performance. They make you think about how you feel, and you're not supposed to think, you're supposed to be so well prepared that you slide into the Zone and perform with grace and purpose. Not possible if your mind is on other things.

Of course, Cleaners are still human, and like everyone else they feel the same excitement and anxiety and nerves before a big event. But the difference between Cleaners and everyone else is their ability to control those feelings, instead of allowing those feelings to control them. Even Michael used to say he had butterflies before a big game. "Get 'em all going in the same direction," I'd tell him. They're not going away, but now you're controlling how you feel about them, instead of allowing them to make you feel nervous. Energy instead of emotion. Big difference.

A Cleaner thinks, If I'm feeling nervous, how the fuck are *they* feeling? They have to deal with *me.*

I want you in a routine, and I don't want that routine to vary, whether it's a meaningless preseason exhibition or the championship game of the Finals. Do what you do every day, so you never have to account for your environment or the situation. Everything stays the same. If it's the night before the game, you have to be able to say, "Okay, I've done everything to get myself to this point, I'm ready." And then enjoy the evening with the family or friends or whomever you enjoy being with, doing whatever you enjoy doing. I want you surrounded by supportive people who know what you need and know you can't give a lot back . . . people who understand you can't take all the uncles and cousins to dinner the night before the big game, friends who don't get you involved in their drama. No emotion, no added pressure. Because the minute you start telling yourself and everyone else, "Whoa, big game tomorrow, don't mess with me," you've become emotional. That's the worst thing you can do.

The night before Miami beat Oklahoma City in 2012, I had Dwyane working out in the arena late at night, and his phone was going off every few minutes with teammates texting to say they couldn't sleep, couldn't settle down. I don't want to hear that. Now you're showing the pressure is getting to you, and you're not in control. I guarantee the youngsters on the Thunder sat around playing video games, fearless and oblivious to what it would feel like to lose at that level, because most of them had never before been there. That kind of innocence doesn't last too long, though; the next time around, they won't be able to sleep either.

Think about that intense moment when you're on the top of a roller coaster, right before it sends you into that wild free fall. You know what's coming, you know it's supposed to be scary. Do you scream? Do you panic? Or do you stay calm and fearless because you know you can handle whatever happens next? The difference is what sets you apart from those who give in to the fear and can't control how they feel.

While others are getting heated up, I want you to start cool and stay cool, because anything that starts too hot can only get cold. When you want to preserve food and keep it fresh, what do you do? Refrigerate it. Keep it cool. Make it last longer. As the lights get brighter and the place gets hotter, you should be feeling darker and cooler, pulling deeper inside yourself. This is your Zone, all instinct; you can feel your way in the dark while others have to see and hear and watch what everyone else is doing. You go with what you feel. The people who can get into that space, those are your killers.

Finding your way into the Zone begins with trusting those instincts, and that's where we're going next.

#1. When You're a Cleaner . . .

. . . You know exactly who you are.

A Cooler thinks about what he's supposed to think about.
A Closer thinks, analyzes, and eventually he acts.
A Cleaner doesn't think at all, he just knows.

W e're all born bad.

Sorry, but that's the truth. Born bad, taught to be good.

Look, if you're already shaking your head and frowning in disagreement, we're not going to get very far. If you want to go somewhere new, you have to throw out the tired, old map and stop traveling the same road to the same dead end. I promise, where we're going, you've never been.

Born bad. Taught to be good.

Or if you prefer: born relentless, taught to relent.

Think about it. We're born already wired with the most basic instincts that guarantee our survival: babies don't have to think about their needs, they don't analyze how they feel, they don't plan or decide how to get what they want. They just know, instinctively, that they're hungry or tired or wet or cold or hot . . . and they scream until they get satisfaction. Pure, preverbal, innate demands for immediate results. You can't argue with a baby or try to convince him he's wrong. You can't put your values on him or explain why he can't eat right now. Babies tell everyone how it's going to be, and that's how it is. They follow their instincts, they thrive, they get what they want.

Babies are completely, naturally, insatiably relentless.

Within a couple of years, they're running around and hollering like crazy, making messes and shoving more food in their hair than in their mouths. Why? Because they're two, and that's what their instincts tell them to do.

And then the grown-ups start reading books about the terrible twos and ruin everything.

Be quiet, sit still, don't run around, stop crying, wait your turn, you're going to hurt yourself, just behave . . . why can't you be more like your brother? Be good!

We take all those powerful natural instincts, those instantaneous gut reactions, we chalk them up to bad behavior and do everything possible to shut them down.

What a waste. All that natural energy, drive, intuition, action . . . reduced to a time-out in the corner. From the time you're a toddler to the time you're an adult, you've been taught to be "good." What's wrong with the way you were?

Born relentless, taught to relent.

Can you even remember a time when you weren't being taught limitations and compliance, watching what everyone else was doing, scrutinizing the options, worrying about what others would say? At some point you stopped doing what came naturally and started doing what you were told. You took all your crazy urges and ideas and desires, and you stuffed them down where no one could see.

But right now, right this minute, you know they're still there, in the part of you that you don't show anyone else, the part that refuses to be taught, refuses to conform and behave. That's the dark side of your instinct.

You cannot be great without it.

Picture a lion running wild. He stalks his prey, attacking and killing at will, and then goes in search of his next conquest. That's what his lion instincts tell him to do, he doesn't know anything else. He's not misbehaving, he's not bad, he's being a lion. Now lock him up in the zoo. He lies there all day, quiet and lethargic and well fed. What happened to those powerful instincts? They're still there, deep inside, waiting to be uncaged. Let him out of the zoo and he goes lion again, preying and attacking. Put him back in the cage, he lies down.

Most people are the lion in the cage. Safe, tame, predictable, waiting for something to happen. But for humans, the cage isn't made of glass and steel bars; it's made of bad advice and low self-esteem and bullshit rules and tortured thinking about what you can't do or what you're supposed to do. It's molded around you by a lifetime of overthinking and overanalyzing and worrying about what could go wrong. Stay in the cage long enough, you forget those basic instincts.

But they're there, right now, waiting for you to find the key to the cage so you can finally stop thinking about what you'll do if you ever get out. All that killer instinct is just waiting to attack.

What's stopping you?

Can you be reasonably successful by just following directions and staying within the lines? Sure. That's what most people do. But if we're talking about being elite, if you want to be unstoppable, you have to learn to put aside everything you've been taught, all the restrictions and limitations, the negativity and doubt.

If that sounds complicated and confusing, let me make it simple:

You have to stop thinking.

It's so basic. Are you good at what you do? Maybe even great at what you do? Can you be the best? Yes?

If you said no, I'll give you a moment to change your answer.

Again: Can you be the best?

Of course you can.

Then why are you still questioning your ability to do it?

Quick answer: because at some point, you made something simple into something complicated, and you stopped trusting yourself.

I get frequent calls from athletes who are completely overwhelmed by all the experts and trainers and nutritionists and coaches, everyone throwing so much at them that they lose the natural ability that made them great in the first place. Anyone who has ever taken a golf lesson understands this: you start out with a decent swing, completely natural, and by the time you're done, you have so much to think about you can't remember why you took up golf in the first place. Anytime you take natural instinct and try to change it, you're going to have a problem. You can build on it, add to it, improve it, but you cannot tame it. There's a difference between training and taming. You can train people to reach higher and be better and go further than they would on their own. But taming means training them to be something less. As the boxer Leon Spinks once said when asked what he does for a living, "I knock motherfuckers out." That's it. Simple. You don't mess with it, alter it, teach it to be something different. That's natural instinct. Leave it alone.

Everything you need is already inside you. You are completely wired with instincts and reflexes specifically designed so you can survive and succeed. You don't have to think about using them, they're always working.

Reflexes are easy: If I whip a ball at your face, are you going to stop and think about what to do? No, you catch the ball or duck out of the way, or you get a busted face. At the very least you're going to flinch. If I flick something toward your eyes, you blink. If you touch something hot, you pull your hand away. We're all born with those basic survival skills. You can't teach or unteach

71

them, they're just part of you. You don't have to think about whether those reflexes will come through, they just always do.

That's how I want you to envision instinct. No thinking. Just the gut reaction that comes from being so ready, so prepared, so confident, that there's nothing to think about. If you're driving, and suddenly the car ahead of you slams on its brakes, do you pause to consider all your options or stop to ask for advice? No, you slam on the brakes. No thought, no hesitation. Instant response, based on experience and preparation. If you think, you die. When you just know, you can act.

Whether you're playing a sport or running a business, it's the same concept. You don't need to schedule a meeting to discuss a decision; you just make the decision. Your instincts become so finely tuned that you have a reflexive response that allows you to attack without thinking.

In other words, you're in the Zone.

Go back to that lion stalking his prey. Silent, determined, focused . . . instinctively knowing that whatever the victim does, he has no chance. The lion waits . . . waits . . . waits . . . until that inevitable moment of weakness. Attack. Done. Next. He doesn't have to be shown what to do or how to think. He knows. So do you.

I guarantee when Kobe retires someday, every single story written about him will talk about killer instinct. And they should: he's the ultimate athletic predator. As a competitor, he locks in on his target, and from that moment, nothing can deter him. He doesn't see or hear or feel anything but the desire to conquer; there's nothing in between him and his prey. He craves it, needs it, and like a true cold-blooded killer, he's prepared to attack.

But people talk about killer instinct as if it were a slogan on a T-shirt, a careless cliché used to describe a fierce competitor. TV commentators sit around discussing it as if it were something in the playbook: "So when can we expect to see that killer instinct?" "Oh, it usually kicks in around the fourth quarter!" They have no clue.

Anyone who has actually experienced its raw power knows it can't be summed up in a couple of words. And most people who claim to have killer instinct rarely do, because when you have that kind of power, you don't talk about it. You don't think about it. You just use it.

Tough challenge, to stop thinking about what others tell you to think. Your coach, your boss, your family, teammates, colleagues . . . they're all experts on what you're supposed to be doing, and they rarely hesitate to tell you. Some of the greatest athletes in any sport can't fight the need to overthink. They study all the film, watch the same replays over and over and over, break down every motion to analyze and prepare the right response to different situations. That's a Closer, learning how to react to someone else's action, waiting for the right moment to respond. But what if that moment doesn't arrive? What if the opponent does the unexpected and goes in a different direction?

Now the Closer has lost his feel for the actual game. He's so completely determined to recognize something he saw on film, waiting for that specific situation, trying to remember all the right answers. Instead of playing his own game, he's playing the other guy's game. Reacting instead of acting. Overthinking. Overanalyzing. That's how you lose the natural ability that made you great in the first place.

It happens to coaches all the time. Some know all the X's and O's, but they watch so much film that they have no personal perspective of what's actually happening on the floor. They can tell you every nuance of what they're seeing on the video, but when a real game gets out of hand, it's as if they're playing Xbox without a controller. No video to rely on, no instincts, no chance for success.

When you become too focused on what's going on around you, you lose touch with what's going on deep inside you. Those are the guys who are perfect in practice, but blow it when it counts. They can't find the Zone, they're distracted by their own thought process, and they don't trust themselves. They're thinking about everything that can go wrong, thinking about what everyone else is doing, thinking instead of knowing, without a doubt, *I got this.*

Michael was the master of not thinking. Before every game, the Bulls' coaching staff would have a team meeting, go over the game plan, talk about the opponent and what to expect. They'd hand out a sheet with plays, basic information, just something for the players to review. Michael would get up, grab the sheet, and go in the other room. Every time. He didn't want to hear what everyone was supposed to do, he already knew it. What are you going to teach him at that moment? Absolutely nothing. If there *was* something he needed to know, he knew it long before you did. He knew way in advance what he had to learn, and how to learn it; he sure as hell wasn't going to wait for game time to find out. His mastery of the game was so flawless it didn't matter what was coming at him, he was ready.

Like all Cleaners, he didn't study the competition, he made the competition study him. Other guys sat there analyzing and contemplating what might happen; he didn't have to. He knew his skills and knowledge were so finely tuned that he could dominate any situation; he worked so long and hard that his body and mind reflexively knew what to do at all times. With Michael, everything became automatic; he repeated those same movements over and over until he didn't have to think about anything, he only had to let those instincts take over.

The greats never stop learning. Instinct and talent without technique just makes you reckless, like a teenager driving a powerful, high-performance vehicle. Instinct is raw clay that can be shaped into a masterpiece, if you develop skills that match your talent. That can only come from learning everything there is to know about what you do.

But real learning doesn't mean clinging to the lessons. It means absorbing everything you can and then trusting yourself to use what you know instantaneously, without thinking. Instinctive, not impulsive . . . quick, not hurried. Knowing without a doubt that all the hours of work have created an unstoppable internal resource you can draw on in any situation. Having the maturity and experience to know who you are and how you got to the top, and the mental toughness to stay there.

That was Kobe, as the oldest player on the USA basketball team at the 2012 Olympics in London. Surrounded by superstars much younger than his thirty-three years—they were calling him OG, as in "Original Gangster"—he was asked by reporters if he could learn anything from the younger guys.

No.

You know everything? asked a reporter.

"I don't know if I know it all," he said, "but I know more than they do."

When you're willing to hit the gym three times a day to take shots and work on every detail of your game as Kobe does, you're pretty much ready for anything. He watches a ton of video, breaks down every shot . . . but he also works relentlessly on what he learns from that video. That's a Cleaner, not just learning but taking what you've learned and creating ways to improve on it. Every action becomes instinctive if you're willing to put the time and sweat into building your arsenal of spontaneous responses. Especially for a veteran player, who knows his maturity and experience and seasoned instinct are priceless compared to that of a kid with fresh legs and a ten-cent head.

You want to see raw Cleaner instinct? Find a video of Larry Bird in the 1988 All-Star Game Three-Point Contest against Dale Ellis. Bird had won the competition the two previous years and was coming back to defend his title, and he made sure there was no doubt he was there to win: "Who's finishing second?" he asked the other players in the locker room. It wouldn't be him. After every shot, as soon as the ball left his fingertips, he turned back to the rack to get the next ball. Never watched a single shot after it left his hand. Some went in, some clanged off the rim, but he never looked. He was already halfway off the court headed back to the bench by the time the winning ball went in; he never even took off his warm-up shirt. All instinct. He didn't have to wait to see what would happen. He already knew.

Stop waiting to be taught something you already know. How many millions of diet and exercise books are sold every year? I promise you, every single person who picks up one of those books already knows the answer: eat healthier and move your body. You can eat these calories or those calories, you can move this way or that way, but the result is the same, and you already know that. You bought that book already knowing what you had to do, you were just waiting for someone to tell you. Again. And instead of just making the decision to eat healthier and move more—for a lifetime, not just for twenty-one days or five hours a month or whatever the trend prescribes—you sat down with a book to analyze the situation. Trust me: no one ever lost weight sitting on the couch with a book.

I'm not telling you to stop searching for answers. But learn about yourself, and then trust what you know so you can build on what you already have. It's not a science. Instinct is the opposite of science: research tells you what others have learned, instinct tells you what *you* have learned. Science studies other people. Instinct is all about you. Are you willing to base your decisions and actions on research done by and about people you don't know, whose best advice is to tell you to change? Who knows you better than you know yourself?

Oprah once said, "Every right decision I've ever made has come from my gut, and every wrong decision I've ever made was a result of me not listening." Exactly. Of course, she also spent twenty-five years doing a show for people who preferred listening to her instead of listening to their own gut, as she told them whom they should believe and what they should do and how they should change. Every day, millions of people showed up to hear someone tell them what they were doing wrong, so they could receive instructions on how to live according to someone else's standards.

I wonder if any of those people came away understanding this:

People don't change. You can make millions of dollars or lose millions of dollars, you can get a promotion or lose your job, gain forty pounds or lose forty pounds . . . but you're still the same person. Exactly the same. You can change environments and spouses and careers . . . you're still the same person. No matter what you try, it's a temporary deal; sooner or later, you're going back to your natural self.

Remember my undelivered note to Dwyane? "In order to have what you really want, you must first be who you really are."

That's a Cleaner. When you look inside, you see what's real. When you look on the outside, you can only see images and what people want you to see, a manipulated picture of the truth. Ask yourself, what would it feel like to just let go of all the external pressure and expectations and just be yourself?

I know you're thinking, "It's not that easy." Well, it doesn't have to be easy. If it were easy, everyone would do it. Lots of people start things; few are able to finish. Why? They don't trust themselves to get to the end. They start thinking about everything that could go wrong, second-guessing their choices, listening to others instead of listening to themselves. Anyone can have a great idea . . . it's what you do with the thought that defines you. In a Cooler, an idea will travel from his brain to his mouth—he has to talk about it, discuss it, share it with others for feedback and approval. In a Closer, it travels farther down toward his gut, but instead is diverted toward his heart, where it becomes slowed down by emotion and more thought. In a Cleaner, though, a thought moves straight to the gut, where instinct takes over and puts it into immediate action.

That's the ultimate difference between a Closer and a Cleaner, by the way. A Closer thinks about what he wants; a Cleaner feels it. A Closer tells his heart what he wants the outcome to be; a Cleaner's heart decides on its own, he never has to think about it. Total confidence in his gut. The difference is that millisecond of pause between thinking, "I can do this," and not having to think anything at all.

When you're great, you trust your instincts. When you're unstoppable, your instincts trust you.

Instinct is what tells you how to finish the fight. When you're listening to a mess of external directions, you're going to end up trying a million little things, without complete confidence that any of them will work. But when you're trusting yourself, you have the focus and efficiency to pinpoint the one big move that will do the job. Think about a boxer, who can go around and around in the ring, ready for anything, until suddenly he seizes the moment he's been waiting for. No wasted motion, no panic, no room for error. He's played the moment in his mind so many times, he's so prepared, he doesn't have to think about it. He knows exactly what to do. That's instinct.

Believe what you know about yourself. When I decided to get a degree in kinesiology, everyone said, "Oh, you're going to be a gym teacher?" No, I'm going to train pro athletes. "You can manage a health club!" No, I'm going to train pro athletes. There is *zero* chance you'll get anywhere if you allow yourself to become paralyzed by soft excuses and countless reasons why you'll never get to where you want to be. Trust your gut to navigate the hard road to get there. The satisfaction and sense of achievement will blow your mind when you finally arrive, knowing you arrived on your own with only your instincts to guide you.

Stop thinking. Stop waiting. You already know what to do.

But instinct is only half the formula; you can't be a relentless competitor without a trip to the dark side, and that's where we're going next.

#1. WHEN YOU'RE
A CLEANER . . .

. . . You have a dark side that refuses to be taught to be good.

A Cooler tries to fight his dark side and loses.
A Closer acknowledges his dark side but isn't able to control it.
A Cleaner harnesses his dark side into raw, controlled power.

You know the story of Dr. Jekyll and Mr. Hyde? A respected, upstanding doctor discovers a potion that temporarily turns him into a dark, sinister predator, and for a while he finds he enjoys being free from fear and morality and emotions, not caring about anyone or anything. For the first time in his life, he does what he feels, not what he's been taught.

Jekyll lives quietly by the rules; Hyde acts on impulse and instinct; he exists only in Jekyll's Zone. Hyde does whatever he wants and doesn't care about consequences or whom he has to destroy in the process.

It's the same guy, same inborn urges, but they can only be unleashed when Jekyll becomes Hyde. Jekyll lives in the light, Hyde exists in the dark, and those instincts can only come out when that dark side is allowed to surface.

That's what we're talking about here—a transformation into your alter ego, your dark side, becoming who you really are, who your instincts drive you to be. Of course, Hyde was a psychopath, and I'm not suggesting you go that far off the rails. But if you want to climb out of your rut and get up to the next level, you have to leave your baggage behind. It's Superman shedding "mild-mannered" Clark Kent's suit and glasses, the Incredible Hulk going green, Batman putting on the cape, the Wolf-man howling at the moon. It's the ability to voluntarily or involuntarily drop all the bullshit and inhibitions and allow yourself to just do what you do, the way you want to do it, performing instinctively at the most extraordinary level. No fear, no limitation. Just action and results.

Remember where we started the discussion on instinct? Born bad, taught to be good?

Welcome to your dark side.

Deep inside you, there's an undeniable force driving your actions, the part of you that refuses to be ordinary, the piece that stays raw and untamed. Not just instinct, but killer instinct. The kind you keep in the dark, where you crave things you don't talk about. And you don't care how it comes across to others because you know this is who you are, and you wouldn't change if you could.

Which you can't, because no one really changes.

You can try, you can make promises, you can seek help and read books and learn ways to suppress your basic nature, but the real person inside you stays the same. It has to. That's who you *are*. It's not bad, it's not good, it's just your natural, untamed instinct telling you what it wants, and driving you to get it. Sex, money, fame, power, success . . . whatever you crave.

And before you try to tell me you don't have a dark side, let me promise you, everyone has a dark side.

In your head, right now, think about the things you don't want anyone to know about you. It's okay, no one will know. The secrets you keep, the maneuvers that have helped you along the way, your desires, your greed, your ego . . . the lust you feel for things you're not supposed to have.

That's your dark side. You need it. Because if you haven't figured it out by now, it's the essential link to getting into the Zone, and achieving what you want.

Fact: I've known a lot of very successful, highly driven individuals, and without exception every single one has a dark side. Their dominance and ability to go off the charts are all driven by something deep and intense; it fuels and sustains them. The fire to prove greatness, sexual energy, insecurity . . . it's something different in every person, but it's all about going to that side of yourself that no one else can see. Getting rid of the safety net and judgmental opinions that hold most people back. Letting go.

Give me an honest answer: How many leaders in sports/business/Hollywood/politics—the top names in any field—can you name with 100 percent confidence they'll never be involved in a scandal? They don't have to be celebrities, it doesn't even have to be a public scandal. How many powerful people would you trust to never get tangled in some kind of moral/ethical/legal/marital/financial/personal controversy?

That's what I thought. Not too many.

And guess what: that's how they became powerful in the first place. They're not bad people, they're just not content to be upstanding, complacent Jekyll. I know conventional wisdom gives you every reason to stay out of trouble, resist temptation, and live a clean and virtuous life. But being conventional is for those content to be ordinary, and ordinary isn't going to take you to the top.

Every time you hear about one of those people—a politician, CEO, athlete, celebrity—involved in something "scandalous" and you shake your head thinking, "What an idiot," you're looking directly at his dark side. He knew what he was doing, he knew the consequences before he did it, and he did it anyway.

He could have controlled his actions if he wanted to, and he didn't. Why? Because when you're used to winning, you want to keep on winning at *everything*. That relentless drive to control the uncontrollable, to conquer everything in your path . . . that's the dark side driving you to be who you really are. No challenge too great, too intimidating, too dangerous, because you have zero fear of failing. Zero. The satisfaction doesn't come from the risk, it comes from mastering it. *I own this.*

The more you take on, the more powerful you feel.

You don't get to be the best at anything without blistering confidence and an impenetrable shell. You get there by taking huge risks that others won't take, because you rely on your instincts to know which risks aren't risks at all. When you're standing at the edge of the Zone, it's your dark side that drives its seductive finger into your back and whispers, "Go."

The dark side is your fuel, your energy. It excites you, keeps you on the edge, recharges you, fills your tank. It's your one escape, the only thing that takes your mind somewhere else and allows you to blow off steam for a brief time. For some it's sex, especially sex with someone they're not supposed to be with. For others it might be exercise or drinking or golf. It can be an obsessive need to work or gamble or spend a lot of money. Anything that creates a private challenge and tests you to control it before it controls you. It's an addiction as powerful as your addiction to success.

The dark side doesn't have to be sick or evil or criminal; you can be a good person and still have this one part of you that remains untamed. Think about your classic superheroes—Spider-Man, Superman, Batman—they all fought for good, but lived dark lives. The darkness is simply the part of you that doesn't see the light of day, it's all internal until you act on it, and you only act on it in private or with others you trust to keep your secret. I'm talking about those basic instincts and behaviors that are so personal that you're the only one who really knows what's there. From the earliest age, you were taught those things were bad—don't touch, don't look, don't say that—so you stuffed them away and learned you shouldn't want them, couldn't have them. But instead, you just craved them more, until you got frustrated with hiding who you really were, admitted the truth to yourself, and finally did what you had always wanted to do.

Staying safe means being limited, and you can't be limited if you're going to be relentless.

Any time you've had an internal struggle over what you want versus what you know is "right" . . . that's your dark side you're wrestling with. And you can wrestle for a while, but you never win, because the dark side can't be pinned. You can try to control it or contain it, but you can't keep it down. It's always going to get back up and continue fighting to control you instead. Look what happened to poor Dr. Jekyll: he ultimately killed himself when he realized Mr. Hyde—his dark side—was emerging on its own, and he could no longer control the uncontrollable.

A Cleaner controls his urges, not the other way around. The dark side isn't about taking stupid risks and getting in trouble; that would show weakness. You can feel your desires and act on them, or not act on them; your self-control is what distinguishes you from everyone else. You can walk away or hold back whenever you choose. You reach for the bottle because you want a drink, not because you need one. You can have the hottest women, enjoy them all, but never get too involved. You can spend another hour at the blackjack table and leave while you're still ahead. You stay at the office working late, knowing you should be at home.

You watch everyone else stumble over themselves trying to keep up with you.

And then you find the next thing you can win, and the next, and the next, because being relentless is a hunger that never subsides. As soon as a Cleaner achieves success, and the adrenaline rush recedes, he needs more and he gets it. The high of getting that result is so great, it's just too hard to come back to earth. He needs to devour it, over and over, always craving that taste of total and complete satisfaction.

But what happens when that satisfaction can only be achieved infrequently? In sports, you can only win that championship once a year. All that competition, hard work, sacrifice . . . for one shot in an entire year. That's it. Once. If you don't win, it's another whole year. And maybe another.

If you're so intensely wired to attack and win, you can't just turn that on and off, it's who you are, it defines you. Never exhaling. Never satisfied. We're talking about day after day, year after year, getting on top and staying there. Being the best and still wanting to improve. Not just thinking about success, but striving to prove it, prove it, prove it. No days off. What are you going to do instead to satisfy that craving?

A Cleaner has to conquer something else, he's too hungry to wait. Something he can dominate and control, something that keeps him sharp and competitive, so he can keep moving on to his next conquest. So he tries something else, something he can do in solitude to fill that void and satisfy that insatiable competitive urge he can't get any other way, something that allows him to remain in the Zone as a predator, a relentless mastermind with killer instinct.

The ability to show up at the gym every day and do what no one else is willing to do, that comes from the dark side. The drive to get to the top and stay up there, year after year? Dark side. A Cleaner with a strong dark side can succeed at whatever he chooses, and his path is usually determined at an early age, by his family or environment or culture. One way or another, he's going to be the best at something. A positive impact on his life might channel him toward business or athletics; a negative impact might direct him into a life of crime. Really, is there that big a difference between the instincts of a powerful businessman and a powerful crime boss and a powerful athlete? They're all "killers" in their field, driven to be the best, diabolical in their strategy for reeling in and crushing the competition, equally relentless in their desire to win at all costs, and none of their victims sees them coming until it's too late. They're not necessarily killing with guns, they're killing with skill and craft and mental weaponry. They're all brilliant at what they do. And they all share the same objective:

Attack, control, win. Anything to get the end result.

And then they do it all again. And again.

Cleaners go home to detach from the dark side; it's the built-in safety valve. That's why so many men fight to stay in their marriages even after they've been caught doing something they shouldn't have been doing: home is the only safe place they know. Home surrounds you with comfort and security; the force of the dark side comes from somewhere else. You go home to feel safe and loved, you go out to feel excitement. Home is for calm and warmth, out there is for heat. You may not want to admit it, but you can't deny it. The fire in your gut comes from the dark side, and the dark side has no place at the family dinner table.

Cleaners understand this. It's what makes them Cleaners. If you're already a Cleaner, you know what we're talking about, and you probably can't believe we're talking about it.

The dark side has nothing to do with what's happening at home; people try to blame it on that, but they know that's an excuse. It's about how they feel on the inside, and no one—at home or elsewhere—can change that. It's who they are.

So they wear a mask of normalcy, not for their own benefit but to protect those they care about; the face on the mask is the person others want them to be. They know they're not being themselves—the only time you can be 100 percent yourself is when you're connected to your dark side—but they do what they have to, so they can ultimately do what they want to.

And then as soon as they can, they go back to their natural selves. They make no distinction between different parts of their lives, the way they work is the way they live: intense, competitive, driven. There is no way to be relentless and do it any other way. Can you control that intensity when you want to, briefly and appropriately? Sure you can. But you rarely want to. When all you think about is winning, you just want to stay in that Zone where it's dark and cool and it's just you and your thoughts.

And when you have to, you wear the mask.

I don't know if there's a better example than Tiger Woods, whose now-famous dark side led him to become involved with a dozen or so women who were not his wife. Of course, that number of women would be a slow week for some pro athletes, but Tiger had done such a good job of wearing the mask and hiding his dark side that people were just blown away by the revelation that Jekyll was smiling for the camera and making the commercials, and Hyde was handling everything else.

You want to see a guy in the Zone, watch video of Tiger before the scandal; he'd walk onto that course as if it were built for him, and if you got in his way, God help you. All the experts loved talking about his mental toughness, how his father trained him by intentionally dropping clubs and moving the cart during his back-swing, how his mother taught him to get out there and "kill them, take their heart." Raised to be in the Zone, said the analysts.

Then the scandal broke and it was suddenly pretty clear exactly what had put Tiger in the Zone.

Once the story came out, one salacious and painful piece at a time, his career began to deteriorate in every way conceivable. With everyone watching and judging and analyzing every detail of his private life, that dark side evaporated; that kind of energy simply can't survive in the light. It completely loses its power, unless you're willing to stand up and say, "Yeah, so what?" and go right on doing whatever you were doing.

That's how you keep your dark side dark.

But Tiger's situation was made even worse by the pressure he felt to make a public apology, because let's face it, when you're making hundreds of millions of dollars off your image as a clean-cut husband and father, your dark side had better stay in the dark.

I have to be honest. As someone who has known and liked Tiger for a long time, I didn't want to see that apology. I wanted to see him say nothing in public and show up ready to fight another day.

Like my friend and client Charles Barkley, who threw a guy through a plate-glass window in an Orlando nightclub after the jackass threw ice at him. You don't throw ice—or anything else—at Charles and expect to get away with it. After the judge dropped the charges, she asked Charles whether he had learned anything from the experience. "Yes," he said, "I shouldn't have thrown him through the first-floor window. I should have taken him to the third-floor window and finished the job from there."

No apologies.

I wanted to see Tiger handle his situation with that kind of confidence. He built this intimidating reputation of being a killer on the golf course; I didn't want to see him hanging his head. He didn't murder anyone. He stepped out on his wife, it's between him and his family. Worried about losing endorsements? Go win something, they all come running back. I wanted him to go out there and show he was still in command of who he was, still a killer, raising his game even higher to show he was still the guy in charge. There is no better way to intimidate the competition: *I went through all of this, and my game went up? You fuckers have no chance.*

And here's the part that underscores how deep that competitive drive can be: there seemed to be an unspoken competition among other athletes and high-profile celebs to see who could outdo him and *not* get caught. "How the *hell* did he get caught?" they wondered. "I'm *never* getting caught!" And if they did, the game would then be to prove they could still perform at the same level and not miss a step, unlike Tiger, who fell way off his game. Another challenge to win, something new to dominate.

Watch this, I control it all, it doesn't control me.

I own this.

Some years ago I knew of a player who decided to challenge his ability to perform after he'd had a couple beers. He'd drink half a six-pack at halftime just so he could go back onto the court and tell the guy across from him, "I just slammed down three beers and I'm still gonna kick your ass." And he would, so that challenge soon became boring. Over the season, he got a couple of his teammates in on the game, to test who could drink the most beers at halftime and still play the best. One day they'd try two beers, another time three beers, four beers . . . they'd keep raising the bar until two of the guys were practically heading for the wrong bench, so the sole survivor (who started the game) could finally say, "Ha! Kicked your ass!"

A ridiculous contest and I'm in no way condoning it, but how else are you going to test what you're capable of if you don't truly challenge your ability under every possible circumstance?

That's what the dark side does: it shuts down the laws of right and wrong and allows you to discover what you're really made of, what you're capable of doing.

I worked with a guy who I believed was drinking too much, and I asked him directly if he had a problem we needed to deal with. Now we had a new challenge. "This is not a problem," he growled at me. "Watch, no drinking for a month." And there was no drinking for a month. Challenge conquered.

Look, I don't care if you want to drink, go ahead. I have no problem with athletes finding ways to relax, they're no different from anyone else in any job. You need to deal with stress? I get it. I've known players to throw back a shot of whatever they needed to relax before a game. And if I make you give it up, you're going to blame me later for messing with what works for you. So go ahead if you have to, if taking that shot is what brings out that dark side and gets you in the Zone.

As long as you stay in control.

Cleaner Law: control your dark side, don't let it control you. Do you want to smoke or do you have to smoke? All that nightlife—do you know when it's time to head home, or is it crushing your game? Do you drink because you like it or because you need it to cope with the pressure you feel? Can you be decent at what you do with an alcohol problem? Probably. But you can't be great.

Cleaners never perform under the influence of anything; they place too much value on their mental state to allow anything to affect their minds and instincts and reflexes. Who's in charge, you or your dark side?

I knew a guy with an addiction for women, who vowed that for one year he wasn't going to screw around. This wasn't an athlete living the celebrity lifestyle, he was a respected business owner with everything to lose, and he didn't care. He made it the whole year, straight and narrow. He was completely miserable, but he was committed to proving he could control himself and thought it might improve his home life (because Cleaners need that stability). Unfortunately, the damage at home was already done, and ultimately so was his marriage. And at the end of the year, his buddies laughed and said, "You just wasted a whole year." But he had to know whether he was controlling his dark side, or it was controlling him.

When tales from the dark side become public, everyone usually sits in judgment and thinks, "He couldn't control himself. Weak." But those aren't Cleaners saying that. Understand this: A Cleaner doesn't *want* to give up the thing you disapprove of. To him, it's not a weakness, it's his strength, his choice. Weakness would mean giving up what he craved because he was afraid of getting caught.

A Cleaner earns his alter ego, his Mr. Hyde. It doesn't blindside him, he goes out and gets it. At some point in his life, something challenged him and made him survive, and the result was his total confidence that whatever happened to him, his instincts would cover his ass and he'd be okay. And somehow he always is. The desire to control anything and everything is so powerful, and his belief in his instincts is so strong, he knows he can't lose.

Be honest: Would you be as successful if you followed all the rules and always behaved and never took chances? No, you'd be just like everyone else, scared about failing and worried about being liked.

Most people can't begin to comprehend the psychological makeup of an individual who is one of the best in the world at what he does, and what he's been through to get there. You can't compare your values and rituals and perspective with his. You just can't. It's not that his mindset is better or worse than yours, it's just unique.

But the bottom line is that he doesn't give a damn what you think about him or his dark side or anything else, because the only pressure he feels is whatever he puts on himself, and as you'll see, he can't ever get enough of it.

#1. When You're a Cleaner . . .

. . . You're not intimidated by pressure, you thrive on it.

A Cooler is never in a situation where he has to be "clutch."
A Closer is "clutch" in high-pressure situations.
A Cleaner is always "clutch."

Let's get this out of the way right now:

There is no such thing as the "clutch gene."

Or if there is, it's not something you should want.

When do you hear that expression? When a guy is under pressure, steps up at the last minute, and makes something miraculous happen.

Everyone goes nuts about how "clutch" the guy is, and for days there's a big discussion about the so-called clutch gene—whatever the hell that is, I still don't know—

and who has it and who doesn't and how you can tell and on and on about this completely false premise.

There is no clutch gene.

There's your predatory instinct that tells you to attack and finish the fight, and there's the readiness to know how and when to do that.

Preparation + opportunity. That's it.

If you're a true competitor, you always feel that pressure to attack and conquer, you thrive on it. You intentionally create situations to jack up the pressure even higher, challenging yourself to prove what you're capable of. You're not waiting for a critical moment to dust off some mythic "gene" to showcase your greatness. You show it in everything you do, every chance you get.

Closers are called Closers for a reason: they show up at the end. They can deliver in a pressure situation because they step up when something is on the line.

For Cleaners, every moment is a pressure situation, and everything is always on the line.

Honestly, if I were you, I'd be insulted if someone said I had a clutch gene. It's not a compliment when people say you step up for the big games. Where were you all the other games? Why weren't you that solid and aggressive and effective all the time?

Look, I get the impact of a guy who sinks the winning shot, or blasts the walk-off home run, or drives down the field and throws the winning TD with two seconds on the clock. I understand the satisfaction of being the guy who gets everyone what they need, when they need it. I get the drama and thrill and intensity of succeeding in that moment, and going home a hero.

But being relentless means constantly working for that result, not just when drama is on the line. Clutch is about the last minute. Relentless is about every minute.

Because if you're content to wait until that last minute, you are way too safe the rest of the time, taking it easy, coasting along in your comfort zone. A lot of guys won't take that last shot, not because they're afraid they'll miss, but because if they make it, they have to *keep* making it. Look at Jeremy Lin: he exploded out of nowhere to play at such a high level for the Knicks, and everyone expected him to stay at that level, which just wasn't going to happen. When you start that high, you have a lot farther to fall and you hit the ground a lot harder from that height. For a lot of guys, it's easier to stay in the comfort zone, close to the ground. Minimal expectations, minimal pressure . . . minimal rewards. But you're safe.

Cleaners crave that height, along with the pressure of staying up there and going higher and higher. As soon as they start relaxing for just a moment, they instantly feel as if they're slacking. If you're a Cleaner, you know that intense rush of needing to control something, attack something, right now. Never, ever, do you go through a day thinking, "That was relaxing." To a Cleaner, relaxing is something weaker people do because they can't handle pressure. Put him in a situation where he's supposed to be relaxed—such as a vacation he didn't really want to take, or a day he doesn't have to work out—and he'll actually become more stressed thinking about what he should have been doing. He'd rather deal with a challenge than put the effort into "unwinding." He likes being wound.

When a Cleaner wants a break from the pressure he puts on himself, he escapes to the dark side. Something else for him to control, a temporary fix that maintains the pressure but allows him to shift his focus from one addiction to another for a while. Instead of working, he reaches for sex. Instead of competing, he goes for the bottle. Instead of obsessing about his finances, he goes to the gym to obsess about his body. Still all about pressure, performance, and pushing the edge of his comfort zone back farther and farther, just to test his own limits. Assuming he has any.

A Cleaner controls the pressure he feels, and he never looks to anyone else to help him control it. This is why I think of LeBron as a Closer, not a Cleaner. When nothing is handed to you—as in Dwyane's case, going to a small high school and a small college—you have to prove yourself every day, over and over; the internal pressure to establish yourself as the best is unrelenting. But when you walk in the door with everyone already telling you you're the best, it's a lot easier to believe. LeBron has been on a pedestal since he was in high school, got the big shoe deal and the billboards before he had done anything, shook up the entire league with the ordeal over The Decision. People who had never watched a basketball game in their lives were asking where LeBron was going to play. Plenty of pressure in that, absolutely. But when you consider he was going to play alongside two other elite players—

Dwyane and Chris Bosh—and was surrounded by an outstanding collection of other players, you realize he had a lot of latitude to spread that pressure around.

You want to make comparisons? Think about Kobe's reign in LA, Michael's years with the Bulls, Dwyane before the Big Three, even Derrick Rose in Chicago: those are guys who at some point looked around at the rest of the league and thought, "I don't want to join you, I want to *beat* you." And when a newcomer shows up, they're all thinking the same thing: "You can join me, but I'm not joining you." When Dwight Howard and Steve Nash joined the Lakers before the 2012–13 season, all eyes were on the dynamic of Kobe and his new teammates. Would they share the starring roles? Was Kobe handing over the leadership role? Were the new Lakers going to get more attention than the originals?

Kobe shut that down right away: "I don't want to get into 'Well, we share,'" he told reporters. "No. It's my team."

I own this.

I understand the desire of great players to play alongside other great players. But use the opportunity to jack up the pressure, not dial it down. Forge that partnership so you can become even more competitive and intense, not so you can share the pressure and take less responsibility.

When LeBron finally got a ring, everyone was saying, "Finally, the pressure is off." Are you kidding me? The pressure just quadrupled. Now you have to get started on doing it again, so you can do it again the year after that. Anyone who is content with one ring and doesn't feel the pressure to earn another needs to retire, effective immediately.

I always felt Michael's legendary trash talking wasn't meant for the other guy; it was another way for him to heighten the pressure he put on himself, because once you've told others how bad you're about to fuck them up, you're gonna have to deliver on that promise.

I tell my guys, "Pressure, pressure, pressure." Most people run from stress. I run to it. Stress keeps you sharp, it challenges you in ways you never imagined and forces you to solve issues and manage situations that send weaker people running for cover. You can't succeed without it. Your level of success is defined by how well you embrace it and manage it.

Because if you don't manage it well, the other guy is waiting to find your weakness, and the moment you show it, he'll attack. Exactly what you should do when someone shows weakness.

During the 2012 NBA Finals, Oklahoma City's Serge Ibaka decided to test how well LeBron was managing the pressure he felt to carry the Heat to a championship. LeBron's mental toughness had been a question for a long time; when he was seriously stressed, he'd start biting his nails and chewing his fingers. When I saw him doing it during the championship series, I turned to ESPN's Stephen A. Smith and said, "He just checked out." The minute he does that, he's gone. This time, fortunately for the Heat, he was able to come back. In the past I've seen him at the free throw line, at home in front of his own fans, giving them the quiet-down arms as if they're being too loud and distracting him. That's how you know the emotion has taken over.

So Ibaka goes right at that emotion and tells the media before Game Four that LeBron can't defend Kevin Durant by himself. Which of course set the media on fire to get a response from LeBron, who said he wasn't going to comment. And then commented at length.

That's a Closer, thinking about it, allowing it to become a distraction, feeling the pressure to prove something. A Cleaner doesn't respond to external pressure, he puts the pressure back on the guy trying to get under his skin by refusing to acknowledge him. Remember, you don't compete with anyone, you make them compete with you. You can control what you put on yourself; you can't control what the other guy puts on you. So you focus only on the internal pressure that drives you. Run to it, embrace it, feel it, so no one else can throw more at you than you've already put on yourself.

Like this: During the 2010 season, the Lakers were playing Orlando, and Matt Barnes was playing for the Magic. The entire game, Barnes did everything possible to antagonize Kobe, including faking the ball at his face, maybe one inch from his nose. Kobe never reacted, never flinched. Not once. After the game, reporters asked how he was able to not respond. His answer? "Why should I?"

I don't want to hear that someone can't "handle pressure." Everyone can handle pressure. Most people choose not to because it's easier to stay safe in the comfort zone. But if you want to be successful, to have that place in the sun, then you have to leave the shade. It's not easy to leave the shade; it's cool and comfortable, compared to the hot discomfort of the sun. But you can't be relentless if you can't take discomfort, and you can't be unstoppable if you only deal with pressure when you have no choice.

Pressure can bust pipes, but it can also make diamonds. If you take the negative view, it will crush you; now you're in an "I can't do this" frame of mind. But the positive view is that pressure is a challenge that will define you; it gives you the opportunity to see how much you can take, how hard you can go. Everyone wants to cut back on stress, because stress kills. I say bullshit. Stress is what brings you to life. Let it motivate you, make you work harder. Use it, don't run from it. When it makes you uncomfortable, so what? The payoff is worth it. Work through the discomfort, you'll survive. And then go back for more.

Of course, you have to be able to recognize the difference between stress that can bring great results, and stress you create yourself that just causes chaos. Showing up unprepared, not putting in the work, blowing off commitments and obligations . . . that's the stuff that creates pointless stress. You had the option to manage those things before they turned into negative situations. But when you're faced with the stress of great challenges set before you—making the team, working for a raise, finishing a job, winning a championship—undeniable gifts are buried under all that pressure. Not everyone gets the opportunity to be stressed by the potential to achieve exceptional things.

But you have to keep that pressure turned up all the time, not just when you need to take it up a notch. In my business, I start to see guys slipping away around March, when they start thinking about the playoffs. The constant pressure starts taking a toll; the mental and physical fatigue starts to become a factor. They get lazy at practice, they stop putting in the extra work, and inevitably it starts to affect their whole game. They just hit the wall.

And what kills me is that the guys who quit first aren't the leaders with all the pressure on them; it's the other guys that can't stay engaged all season. The leaders don't have the luxury of checking out. It's one thing when you're in an individual sport—if you quit, you quit on yourself. With a team sport, you have a lot of other people relying on you, and you know that every day someone is mentally taking the day off, so you're going to have to cover for him. But you don't know who it's going to be—who's showing up to play, who's not really showing up at all—until you're right there in the middle of the situation. So there's even more pressure to figure out what you're working with.

And eventually, even the leaders start to drift.

At that point, I'll sit down with my guys and say, "Guess what, your team isn't even in the playoffs yet. Wake the hell up. Because here's what you get if you make the playoffs and stay in the playoffs: a ring, and all the glory that goes along with it. And here's what you get if you don't make the playoffs: you get to go home.

"You had a great season? So what? Those other guys had great seasons, they're still playing, and you're not. It's not enough to get to the top. You have to stay there. Feel that pressure, and fight to stay there. You have to work for that. It's not owed to you."

That's how you know when the great ones are finally done: they no longer want to keep fighting that fight. They know what they've accomplished, and they make the choice to stop cranking up the pressure. And it's always a choice, completely in their control. I saw it in Michael when he went to play in Washington; the psychological aspect of being Michael Jordan, what that represented to so many people around the world, craving that pressure and turning it into diamonds every day, year after year, constantly striving to be better than the best, when you're already the best . . . eventually you just have to say, "Enough. This is who I'm going to be now." The fire was still there, but not that desire to make it hotter and hotter. And he was still the only player ever over the age of forty to score more than 50 points in a game. Even then, he'd still do something to thrill the crowd, his way of saying, "Just because I don't doesn't mean I can't," letting the next opponent know he was still there to be dealt with. He still craved the pressure, still had fun finding ways to crush the other guy. No question in my mind he could have kept playing.

When you deal with stress all the time, it becomes second nature. It's still not easy or effortless, but you handle things without panicking because you have experience in accepting the rigors of complex challenges. When you never have to take on anything harder than your daily routine, when you shy away from anything that rocks your sense of safety and control, you're much more likely to fall apart at the first twinge of pressure.

Cleaners never feel external pressure; they only believe what's inside them. You can criticize, analyze, demonize a Cleaner, but he's still only going to feel pressure from within. He knows what he's doing right, and what he's doing wrong. He does not care what you think. He steps out of his comfort zone and challenges himself to get to the next level.

It all goes back to confidence. When you're challenged, do you bring the pressure, or do you let the other guy push you into a corner? Do you feel trapped like a rat or do you attack first? Do you pull back, afraid of the fight, or do you make the other guy get in the mud with you? Wounds heal, scars don't; those are your combat medals. In the MJ days, we'd say, "Go get some on ya." Go get dirty.

#1. When You're a Cleaner . . .

. . . When everyone is hitting the "In Case of Emergency" button, they're all looking for you.

A Cooler waits for you to tell him the plan.

A Closer works on the plan, studies it, memorizes it, and knows exactly what he has to do.

A Cleaner doesn't want a specific plan; he wants every possible option available to him at all times.

Every season, it's a lock that on the first day of October training camp, my phone will start blowing up with calls and texts from players who spent the summer living the NBA lifestyle and suddenly realized, "Damn, I forgot to get ready to play." Or I get the agents and the

GMs calling in a panic because they finally figured out their main guy didn't do the work over the summer, and now they're all going to have to figure it out on the fly.

In case of emergency, break glass. By the time I get that call, I know plenty of others have tried and failed to get control, and they're out of answers and options. If you're a Cleaner, you know what I mean: everyone else wanted to handle the situation themselves, and when they finally realized they couldn't, they all came looking for you. And in most cases, you knew it was coming, you just watched and waited. Now everyone is watching you to see how you're going to manage a situation that seems unmanageable. And you'd better be able to figure it out fast.

When I arrived in Miami to help Dwyane during the 2012 Finals, I knew two things: I was walking into a situation that was already damaged, and I was supposed to do what no one else had been able to do. Dwyane's main concern was whether I could help his injured knee in such a short window of time, or if was too late to do anything for the remainder of the playoffs; the Heat were already headed into Game Three. I was honest: Here's what I can and can't do. You're going to need surgery after the season. If you're looking for me to help you avoid the surgery, it's not going to happen. But can I get you through a seven-game series? Absolutely. Will you feel better? Yes, you will definitely feel better.

I am 100 percent certain that if you bring me into any situation, I'm going to have a positive impact on you. There's no way I'm going to show up and not be prepared, and not have something to offer you. If you're willing to listen to what I'm asking you, tell me what I need to know, and follow what I say, you're going to have some improvement.

If that sounds like arrogant swagger, fine with me. I'm confident in what I do because I know whatever happens, I'm going to adjust and keep rolling. Not everything works the first time, sometimes it doesn't work at all. But there's a difference between confidence and cockiness: confidence means recognizing something isn't working and having the flexibility and knowledge to make adjustments; cockiness is the inability to admit when something isn't working, and repeating the same mistakes over and over because you stubbornly can't admit you're wrong.

When I talk to a team's training staff about one of my clients, telling them what we've been doing and what they have to do to keep our guy healthy, at some point I'm probably going to hear, "Right, sounds great, but that's not really how we do it here." Well, yeah, if that *were* how you did it, I wouldn't be here. But I *am* here, and now you have to adapt to what I'm telling you works for him.

My job is no different from that of the corporate troubleshooter who comes in to turn around a troubled business, or a general manager hired to put together a winning team. When what you're doing isn't working, find someone who can make it work. And then let him do it.

That's the Cleaner's job.

Not everyone wants that job. It leaves you completely exposed and open to all kinds of criticism and scrutiny. But it never occurred to me that if Dwyane's knee worsened, or if he had a couple of bad games, it would somehow reflect on me, that people would say, "Grover couldn't get it done." I just don't think that way. It would certainly have been easier to stay where I was, working with Kobe in Los Angeles, getting ready for the Olympics. I could just have given Dwyane some advice and told him we'd get together over the summer. I hadn't worked closely with him for two seasons, so basically, I had three hours to learn about the last two years to get through the next five days before looking ahead to the next two seasons. But when I see a challenge that everyone else has failed to own, I'm going to own it.

Because when the series ended, Dwyane was holding up that trophy, and that's the payoff no words can describe. You take the risk to taste that greatness.

A Cooler takes no risks.
A Closer takes risks when he can prepare in advance and knows the consequences of failing are minimal.
Nothing feels risky to a Cleaner; whatever happens, he'll know what to do.

Picture a military operation with a specific tactical strategy: go into that building, make sure it's empty, go out the red door and into the waiting truck in back before the building blows up. You do exactly as ordered, everything goes according to plan . . . until you get to the red door. Locked. No other exit. Now what? Panic? Those ten seconds you spend panicking might be your last. A Closer will feel fear first, then fumble for an option. But a Cleaner will instantly feel his survival instincts kick in, giving him a rush of options, and he knows one of them will work because he's already considered thirty variables before going into the building. (A Cooler would never be given that kind of assignment, so we don't even have to address him here.)

If you're a Cleaner, you know that feeling, and you've likely been in that kind of situation when everyone else is freaking out and you just know what to do. You don't even know *how* you know, you just know. I'm not talking about "winging it" or making it up as you go. I'm talking about being so prepared, with so many options and so much experience, that you're truly ready for anything.

Some people know without a doubt they'll be okay no matter what happens. Others choke as soon as things go wrong. You see it in sports all the time: a figure skater falls, a quarterback throws a pick, a pitcher gives up a grand slam. Everything that happens after that moment goes one of two ways: the athlete either immediately turns it around and comes back to perform at an insanely high level, or he can't recover and it gets worse from there.

Why? Same talent, same routine they've gone through a thousand times. Why can some adapt to an unexpected twist, and others completely fall apart?

It's not just a sports phenomenon; you can look all around you and recognize people who can handle anything, and others who can handle nothing. What makes the difference?

Few people have the ability to adapt on the fly and make quick adjustments that work. You can plan and prepare for ten different scenarios, be completely ready for every variable you anticipated . . . and you can be sure there will be an eleventh scenario you never saw coming. Most people are ready for one scenario, they can't even envision ten; they're completely paralyzed by all the possible variables, and when one thing goes wrong, they can't adjust.

You can practice the same shot over and over and over, until you can do it blindfolded. Great, now can you do it if I hit you with a sandbag while you shoot? Can you focus if I blast horrible music or scream in your face? When you always go according to plan, you get robotic and lose that innate ability to know what to do when plans suddenly change, when you're confronted by the unexpected. But a Cleaner can take that same plan, and when something goes off the rails, his instincts immediately take over and he adapts. Doesn't think about it, doesn't need to be told, he just knows.

That's the trademark of a dangerous competitor: he doesn't have to know what's coming because whatever you show him, he's ready. No fear of failure.

That's not about the myth of "positive thinking"; it's about the hard work and preparation that go into knowing everything there is to know, letting go of your fears and insecurities, and trusting your ability to handle any situation.

I'm not saying you can't think about what you have to do, but do your thinking and planning in advance, building your reflexes, so you know when your back is against the wall, you've got the right move. You don't accomplish that by obsessing and worrying until you're an emotional mess, unable to sleep or focus on anything else. You prepare yourself by knowing you're ready with the next bullet to fire. You don't ever have to pull the trigger, but you have to know it's locked and loaded and available if you need it.

How quickly can you make that adjustment if you take the wrong step? Can you recognize the mistake and snap it back? You have to be willing to fail if you're going to trust yourself to act from the gut, and then adapt as you go. That's the confidence or swagger that allows you to take risks and know that whatever happens, you'll figure it out. Adapt, and adapt again.

I don't think you can really understand relentlessness until you've faced your worst fears, and you've experienced that internal response telling you what to do. If you think back to the major events in your life, you can probably identify the things that impacted everything else and taught you what you were capable of dealing with.

This is one of the ways I learned: My family came to the United States when I was four, and my father went to work in the basement of a hospital in Chicago, dismembering cadavers. When there was no school and both my parents were working, he'd take me with him; I was five years old the first time I saw my father dismantle a corpse. When I was six, he handed me a bone saw and told me to help. His lesson to me: this is how a man provides for his family.

That's how I learned: you figure it out.

My parents are from India, and they moved to London after they were married; I was born there. My mother was a nurse, and my parents decided she would go to America to work because they wanted a better life for my brother and me. For a year, she lived alone in Chicago and the rest of us remained behind until she and my father finally saved enough for us all to be together.

On the day we arrived in Chicago to be reunited as a family, my dad got a cab at the airport, loaded up all our bags and possessions, and we headed toward the city. But a few miles from our destination, he suddenly told the cab to stop. We got out, unloaded all the bags, and started walking, just two little boys who had no idea what was going on, and our dad making it sound as if we were on this great adventure, seeing the city on foot. But the truth was, he didn't have enough money to go any farther by cab. So we carried the bags and walked. He was a dad in a new country with two little boys and no money in his pocket.

Figure it out, I learned.

Even today, he still has that instinctive ability to know whatever he does, it's going to work, and he passed that along to me. Total Cleaner. He came from nothing, asked for nothing, and knew he could make it on his own.

Being relentless means having the courage to say, "I'm going for this, and if I'm wrong, I'll make a change and I'll still be fine." You can't control or anticipate every obstacle that might block your path. You can only control your response, and your ability to navigate the unpredictable. Whatever happens, you have the smarts and skills to figure it out and arrive at the outcome you wanted in the first place.

And when I say "figure it out," I don't mean thinking about it for a week and asking everyone you know what they think. I mean immediately, instinctively, hearing that voice inside saying, "This way!" And you go.

Of course, it's not possible to be 100 percent accurate and successful all the time; instinct doesn't recognize nuance and detail, it just flashes at you and allows your skill to take over, so it's entirely possible to rely on instinct and still make the wrong decision. You see that happen in game situations all the time: a batter swings at a pitch that looks good, just before it curves away from him, a lineman anticipates the snap and jumps offside. Perfect example: In Game Four of the 2012 NBA Finals, with seventeen seconds on the clock, five seconds on the shot clock, and the Thunder down by 3, Russell Westbrook intentionally fouled Miami's Mario Chalmers, not recognizing it was a "Don't foul!" situation. If he had thought about it, he wouldn't have committed the foul. But his instincts told him to foul. And you have to take into account he's young, had never been in that situation before, he's thinking about seventeen seconds on the clock, not five seconds on the shot clock. Chalmers then made two free throws, giving Miami a 5-point lead, and the Thunder lost.

Should Westbrook have known better? Of course. But that flash tells me what kind of player he is, and in the long run he's going to benefit from that flash more often than not. Because if the alternative is waiting and thinking and being too timid to snap into action out of fear you'll blow it, you're going to fail anyway. As hockey great (and Cleaner) Wayne Gretzky said, "You miss one hundred percent of the shots you don't take."

You want to know a true sign of a Cleaner? He feels no pressure when he screws up and has no problem admitting when he's wrong and shouldering the blame: When a Cooler makes a mistake, he'll give you a lot of excuses but no solutions. When a Closer makes a mistake, he finds someone else to blame. When a Cleaner makes a mistake, he can look you in the eye and say, "I fucked up."

That's it. Confident, simple, factual, no explanation. You made a mistake? Fine. Don't explain it to me for an hour. The truth is one sentence, I don't need a long story. You tell me you messed up, take responsibility . . . now you've gained my trust. As soon as you start giving me reasons and rationalizations, I know you have something to hide, and you're not ready to take ownership. Save us both the time. You fucked up. Say it. There is not a faster way to alleviate pressure. "Man, I fucked up." Okay. There's no comeback for that, you owned it. Now fix it. You can't fix something unless you admit it.

People think admitting mistakes creates more pressure because now they're to blame for something. False. The ability to put your hands up and say, "Yep, my fault," is the greatest way to *stop* the pressure. Now you only have one objective: resolve the issue. As long as you continue to deny responsibility, you have the added burden of covering your mistake, and you know the truth will eventually come out anyway. Why bother prolonging the drama? You screwed up, admit it.

Cleaners will just get in your face and announce that you fucked up; they're completely desensitized to criticism and blame, and they expect you to be the same. To you it feels like an attack; to them, it feels like a couple of guys working out a situation. Their confidence level is so high they have no problem admitting when something has gone wrong. They know they can make it right. No problem.

I've made tons of mistakes, I'm going to make plenty more. But I never think of them as failures. Failure to me is when you bring other people into it, when you're looking for an out instead of accepting your own mistake and planning a route to resolving the issue. Once you start blaming others, you're admitting you had no control over the situation. And without that control, you can't create a solution.

Are there times when you truly have no control? Absolutely. But at that point, it's on you to figure out how to take charge and navigate forward. Otherwise, you're allowing external pressure to dictate the outcome. Create your own pressure to succeed, don't allow others to create it for you. Have the confidence to trust that you can handle anything.

When you can laugh at yourself and not take every setback seriously, that's confidence. On the other hand, when someone says something to you that you don't like or you don't want to hear, and you allow it to put pressure on you, even for a moment, that's a confidence problem. When you're confident, you don't care about what others think; you can take your mistakes seriously but still laugh because you know you can and will do better. Cleaners always have the confidence to know they'll get it right. Accept the consequences and move on.

If I spend every day working with a guy and he goes out and has a lousy game, I don't blame him for the lousy game. I know everyone else is blaming him for the lousy game, but I'm wondering if something we did in the gym affected his shot. That's my job; the pressure is on me to ensure he doesn't have two lousy games. It would be easy to shrug it off—most people would—but if you want to be the best, you never have the luxury of shrugging off a bad performance. You face it, fix it, and prepare to do better next time.

People ask me if I ever get nervous during games. I get nervous when my guys do stupid things, make bonehead plays, or blow something we worked on, moments that make you think, "You gotta be kidding me. How could you *do* that?" Because now I have to ask myself if maybe I didn't do something right, maybe I didn't explain something properly. I told one of my guys recently we had to get his eyes checked. "For what?" he said. "I got perfect vision." Man, get your fucking eyes checked, okay? You turned the ball over so much this year, I just want to know if there's a vision problem, so we can address it. Is it a depth problem? Let's just find out. If I'm wrong,

I'm wrong. I might be wrong, let's find out. Just help me know if I'm not teaching you right, or you're not seeing it right.

When I work with Kobe, we try a lot of new things because he's so dedicated to his workouts that we have time and latitude to experiment with different ideas. So when we've worked on something new and he has a rough game, I don't look to him and wonder what he did wrong. I put the pressure on myself to figure out what I need to do differently for him. I have to ask if we did something to affect his shot, maybe one of the exercises is affecting his movement in a certain way. . . . I need to compensate for all of that. My responsibility, not his.

When I spent those few days with Dwyane during the playoffs, we did so much in a short time, there was no chance to really test how his body was going to react. A lot of his muscles had shut down, and now they were suddenly working again, so he was moving at a faster pace, more gracefully, more explosively. And when you've been working at one speed, and suddenly you can move a lot faster, your timing is going to be jacked.

But it didn't even hit me that I needed to explain that to him, until the minute he started moving in Game Three and he immediately turned the ball over because his timing was off. And I just thought, "Damn, I didn't mention that to him." I realize 99.9 percent of people watching had no idea that was a factor in a game, but to me, it was all my responsibility, and I blew it. My fault. I know it doesn't sound like a big deal, but to me, it was a very big deal because I missed something I shouldn't have missed.

Yes, he had a good game and Miami won, but maybe he could have played even better and they could have won by more.

And it would have been easy for me to say nothing about it because he had no idea what had happened; he just knew he turned the ball over. But that's not me: when I'm wrong, I'll tell you. My mistake, my miscalculation, and I told him that after the game. That's internal pressure at work, getting on yourself for something no one else would even notice and challenging yourself to get it right. Not because you have to, but because you want to.

Have the confidence to say when you've screwed up, and people will respect you for it.

If you did it, own it. If you said it, stand by it. Not just the mistakes, but all your decisions and choices. That's your reputation. Make it count. If you want your opinions to have value, you have to be willing to put them out there and mean what you say. Two things you can't let anyone take from you: you can't let them take away your reputation, and you can't let them take away your balls. That means accepting the pressure of taking responsibility for everything you say and do.

Maturity, experience, practice . . . the more educated you become, the more you heighten your ability to adapt to situations because experience gives you a better understanding of nuance, the tiny details no one else would think of or recognize as important. I'm not talking about accepting a single set of rules, taking what one person thinks and making it your own; I want you to put together your own composite of learning, taking what you know and believe, adding what others have taught you, combining everything you've learned, and creating your own set of beliefs. Not one directive that was set by someone else, but establishing your own.

When you're young, you have one speed—fast. As you mature, you learn to vary your speed based on the situation: you know when to go slow, when to go full out. Here's the example I give my players: Two bulls stand on top of a hill, a father and a son, looking down on a field of cows below. The son can't wait: "Come on, let's go, we gotta run down and get some of those cows!" And the father looks at him slowly, wisely, and says, "No, let's walk down and get *all* the cows." Instinct, not impulse.

The most successful people are those with the instincts to respond quickly to anything, without having to go back to the drawing board, watch more film, schedule a meeting, schedule a meeting to discuss what will be discussed at the meeting, or do any of the other countless things people do to put off making a decision. A couple years ago I was doing a youth camp for one of the big NBA sponsors, along with one of my players. They were expecting five hundred kids. Two thousand showed up. Everyone went into a panic: not enough stations, nowhere to put everyone, how did this happen, who's to blame . . . Stop. Slow down. What do we have, what do we need? Give me ten minutes. I threw out the original plan, devised a new one. We'll do it this way. Of course there's always someone who can't adapt, still clinging to the original failed plan, stammering, "But . . . but . . . we were going to do this and that and . . ." No. We're going this way. Conversation over. Cleaned. That's what Cleaners do, they ignore the panicking and complaining, they clean up the problem and they make it work.

A Closer will adjust himself to the situation; a Cleaner adjusts the situation to himself. A Closer has to know what he's going to do. A Cleaner doesn't; he never wants to be locked in to one plan. He'll know the original plan, and he'll follow it if it feels right to him, but his skills and intuition are so great that he'll usually improvise as he goes; he can't help it. He just goes with the flow of the action, and wherever his instincts take him, that's what you get.

#1. When You're a Cleaner . . .

. . . You don't compete with anyone, you find your opponent's weakness and you attack.

A Cooler does a good job and waits for a pat on the back.
A Closer does a good job and pats himself on the back.
A Cleaner just does a good job, that's his job.

When you're a Cleaner, there's no such thing as a meaningless game. Doesn't matter if it's the first preseason event or a midseason All-Star Game or the last game in a losing season, a Cleaner shows up to play.

During the 2012 All-Star Game, things got a little intense: Dwyane fouled Kobe, gave him a concussion, and broke his nose. Even for a regular-season game that would have been a lot of damage, but this was the All-Star Game, and a lot of people thought Dwyane was out of line.

That's a Cleaner. He sees a situation, his killer instinct kicks in, and he attacks. *I own this. This is what I do. No hard feelings.*

But this story is about two Cleaners, and after the game, there was Kobe, surrounded by an army of doctors and league officials and team personnel trying to examine him and get him to the hospital. He can barely move, nose busted, head ringing, and he's refusing to go. Why? He wanted to see Dwyane and address the situation.

Eventually, though, we got him to leave, Dwyane apologized the next day, Kobe refused to miss a game, and the story faded away. No hard feelings.

But believe this: When you get two relentless individuals going against each other, that situation can play out for years. They can still be cool with each other, hang out, get along . . . but the Cleaner inside never forgives and never, ever, forgets.

That's how Cleaners compete. They dish it out, they take it, and they make sure everyone else does too.

But not everyone can take it. I have this theory, yet to be disproven, that any player 6'10" or over cannot handle harsh, confrontational criticism. With someone 6'9" or under, you can get in his face and just blast him. But any taller, he'll just lose it and go right into a shell. I think it comes from a lifetime of being stared at and gawked at for being so much bigger than the rest of the population, people pointing and making height jokes, so the tall guys become more sensitive and self-conscious. They're just emotional softies. They can be complete killers in competition, but they're also the guys you have to pat on the back, boost their confidence, and make them feel good about what they're doing. The little guys? You can call them every name imaginable and they keep right on going.

I bring this up to give you an example of how different people respond to competitive smackdowns.

This was back during one of the Bulls' championship runs, and Scottie Pippen was trying to get Luc Longley fired up during the Finals. All the players were together before the game, and Scottie was talking to Luc, who stands 7'2".

"Need you to bring your A game," said Scottie.

And before Luc could respond or even nod, Michael whipped around in front of everyone and said, "Bring your A game? Bring *a* game."

Luc was done. I don't think he scored once. Confidence shot. Goodnight.

Michael didn't know—or didn't care to know—how to psychologically deal with teammates. For all his countless gifts as a player, sensitivity to others was not among them. He was driven to attack, dominate, and conquer in every way. Whatever he had to do, he did it, and he expected the same from every individual around him.

And every day, those teammates had to show up to face him in practice, completely dreading what was ahead, not because practices were hard but because they knew they had to deal with #23 and that legendary mouth.

Every. Fucking. Day. Just absolutely going after each and every guy, pushing, demanding, challenging, abusing, finding every possible way to get under their skins and make them go harder.

Once during the playoffs, on the day after a grueling overtime game, the team was ready to start practice until Michael looked around and noticed one guy was missing. "Where the hell is Burrell?" he barked.

Scott Burrell, a part-time player at best, was in the training room. Michael stormed in there, where poor Scott was on the table getting treatment for an alleged hamstring issue. MJ grabbed the table—with Scott still on it—and completely flipped it over.

"I just played forty-eight fucking minutes last night!" Michael roared. "Everything's killing me, and *you* have a fucking hamstring? Get your fucking ass in the fucking practice now!"

Get on my level, or get the hell out of my way.

When you're the guy at the top, it's on you to pull everyone else up there with you, or everything you've built comes crashing down. Not so easy for a Cleaner who demands excellence of himself and has no tolerance for those who can't or won't rise to that level. Does he dumb himself down so he can fit in, slap people on the back, tell them they're great, and hope everyone can rise together? Or does he stand up there alone, set the example, and make everyone else work harder? The answer seems obvious, but you'd be surprised by how many people don't want to stand alone under the glare of the spotlight, because as soon as you reveal what you're capable of, that's what everyone will expect of you. But when no one realizes how good you are, you don't have to be the guy making miracles and running the show, no one will expect much, and everything you do will seem heroic. Easier that way.

Easier, that is, if you're okay being average.

A lot of gifted people will lower their skills to close the gap between themselves and those around them, so others can feel more confident, involved, and relatively competitive. I've seen Kobe do that briefly when he has to, as a way to bring his teammates into the action and keep them engaged. It can work well depending on the other players, and as soon as Kobe sees his teammates stepping up, he'll revert to his natural game. It's a conscious decision to make the other guys feel as if they were one team, not one superstar surrounded by a second-rate supporting cast.

Michael went the other way and came right out and said it: that's my supporting cast.

His message was clear and unrelenting: Hey, I'm not bringing my game *down* so you can look better; you bring your game *up* so you can look better. He refused to put his own game in the backseat just to give other guys more action, unless you proved to him you could handle the responsibility.

If you ever watched the Jordan-era Bulls, you know this scene: Paxson brings the ball up the middle, kicks it to Michael on the wing, Michael throws it to Cartwright, Cartwright takes the shot, he scores or doesn't. Next possession, same thing, Paxson brings the ball up the middle, kicks it to Michael on the wing, Michael passes to Cart-wright, he scores or doesn't. . . . Okay, Cartwright, you got your two touches, you're done for the game, don't say I didn't give you the fucking ball. Now I gotta go do what I need to do.

During a game, Michael would assess who was and wasn't giving 100 percent and make his own adjustments. He never showed frustration on the court; his body language and demeanor never changed. He'd just say, "You're not playing tonight? That's fine, I'll play for all five of us. You keep it close into the fourth quarter, I'll do the rest." And he'd do it in a way that uplifted everyone else, as if that were the game plan all along.

It's far more typical for stars to get aggravated and emotional when their teammates don't show up, and then everyone falls apart because, as we've discussed, emotions make you weak, and all that emotional energy is completely destructive.

But Michael never showed it inside the lines during a game. He always stayed positive, always had fun out there. *After* the game he was like Genghis Khan: he'd go after your balls and your head and everything in between. But during the game, while he was in that Zone, it was all about taking control, staying cool, and getting that end result.

Before Dennis Rodman was traded by San Antonio to the Bulls in 1995, he would occasionally decide to take a night off, and every time he did, the Spurs would lose. The message: can't win without me. So when he got to Chicago and was eventually hit with an eleven-game suspension for kicking a courtside photographer, he couldn't wait to show that the Bulls couldn't win without him either. Really? On Michael Jordan's team? Every game Rodman missed, Michael and Scottie played as if it were for a championship; there was zero chance Michael was going to allow Rodman the opportunity to say the Bulls needed him to win. And he didn't talk about it behind Rodman's back, he said it straight to his face: your bullshit won't fly here, we will win with you or without you.

Get on my level.

Michael knew who was ready, and whom he could trust. He loved Steve Kerr because Kerr would stand up to him. During a now-legendary training-camp scrimmage, Kerr didn't appreciate something Michael said, snapped at him, and Michael punched him in the face. "It was one of the best things that ever happened to me," Kerr said years later. "I needed to stand up and go back at him. I think I earned some respect." He was right. As soon as practice ended, Michael called him from his car, apologized, and from that point on, Michael knew they could go to battle together.

No one would have imagined that Kerr—a Closer as a player and a total Cleaner in everything he earned after he departed the Bulls, including two more rings with the Spurs, a career in the broadcast booth, and a stint as GM of the Phoenix Suns before returning to his television career—would be the player Michael trusted the most on the team. When Michael needed to make a fast adjustment because he knew he wasn't going to be able to get a shot off on the next play, it was Kerr he'd look for and say, "Steve. Be ready." Not Scottie or Horace or Kukoc; Michael trusted Kerr.

That's a Cleaner, deciding what the Closer will do. A Closer can never be put into the Cleaner's role unless the Cleaner decides that's the best way to go. No way Kerr was taking a last-second shot unless Michael wanted him to. And there's also no way Kerr would have had a second chance if he wasn't successful the first time.

People like to make comparisons between Magic and Michael, but Magic looked for Kareem on the floor. Michael looked for no one. He used to tell the guys at the beginning of the season: I'm going to pass you the ball one time. If you don't do something with it, I'm not throwing it to you again. I can miss a shot on my own, I don't need your help for that. So make something happen, 'cause you're only getting one chance. Earn it.

When a Cleaner puts you in a position to execute, you'd better be prepared. At some point, whether you're in the boardroom or the locker room or anywhere else you want to excel, someone is going to point in your direction and say, "You." It may be an opportunity that lasts a minute, maybe ten minutes, maybe a week or a month. But what you do in that time is going to determine what you're going to do for a long time after. Someone is going to do something the coach or the boss doesn't like, maybe a guy isn't playing well or working hard enough, and you're going to get the chance to take his spot. Will you be ready? Will you have done the work that allows you to step in, fully prepared, and show you should have had that job all along? Have you been finding ways to stay sharp and focused? Because if you do well and impress someone, you're in the system. Now the head guy knows he can go to you, and you've added a weapon to his arsenal going forward. But if you don't do well, you're done. The next guy will get the opportunity you didn't grab. You got your chance, you won't get another.

A Cleaner tells you what he expects and demands you deliver. Dwight Howard tells a great story about calling Kobe just before the start of the Lakers' 2012 preseason, to tell him he was feeling good, that his surgically repaired back was probably at 85 percent. "That's good," said Kobe. "Need you at one hundred percent. Trying to win a ring. Bye." Get on my level, or get out of my way.

Michael forced every one of his teammates to be ready, to play better, harder, stronger, and every one of them ended up with careers they could not duplicate when they were no longer playing with him. You don't have to like it, he said, but you'll like the results. And he was right, they didn't like it. But they *all* elevated their games, they all looked better than they were, and they all got a payday. Even the guys with zero minutes, he made them better too. He took the pressure off everyone and put it all on himself.

And when they eventually had to play without him, either because he left or because they went to other teams, almost all of them returned to their natural skill level, physically and mentally. You'd watch some of them in the post-Bulls era and think, "You gotta be kidding me, what happened to that guy?" Teams were signing ex-Bulls and suddenly realizing, "We paid all that money for *this*?" What happened was Michael. No Michael, no relentless pressure, nobody holding them accountable and demanding unyielding excellence. Some of those guys went on to have outstanding careers in other areas—Steve Kerr and John Paxson, to name a couple—but most of the others couldn't keep themselves at the level they were at when they were playing up to Michael's expectations.

But don't be fooled: a true Cleaner isn't thinking about making you better for your benefit. He's happy for you if you get something out of it, but whatever he's doing, it's for his sake, not yours. His only objective is putting you where he needs you to be so he can get the result he desires.

Look at Miami's 2012 championship season. You can talk all you want about LeBron's stepping up in that final game, but without Dwyane's putting him in that position, it couldn't have happened. Remember, a Closer can take the winning shot, but the Cleaner gets him on the team and makes sure the ball is in his hands when it needs to be there. That sums up Dwyane and LeBron completely: Just as Michael did with his teammates—the Cleaner deciding what a Closer will do—Dwyane knew he had to hold back all season so LeBron could step up. No question about it. That's a Cleaner crafting a plan: If I do this, then he'll do that, and in the end we win. And in Dwyane's case, it was even more genius when you remember he was playing on a severely damaged knee that limited what he could do himself. So he put everyone else in place to do it for him.

Mission accomplished. You don't question the methods, you just look for the results.

Dwyane was the mastermind of that team, and LeBron played the role he was sent to play. I just can't look at it any other way. Dwyane was like the father lion, LeBron was the baby lion, and the baby lion knew that whatever he did, he always had the father lion right there, just in case. And when Dad needed to step in and protect the family, he did, and the baby went right on doing whatever he was supposed to do. You take Dwyane off that team, they can't win that championship. It doesn't matter how skilled LeBron is; without Dwyane's leadership the 2012 "Big Three" Heat would have been just another team loaded with talent and no rings.

But you'll never hear Dwyane say any of that or take any credit because, in his mind, that was his job. A great leader knows the best way to get people to raise their performance is to put them where they can truly excel, not just where you want them to excel. Cleaners don't block others from reaching the top with them, if they're capable and ready. And as LeBron evolves as a leader and potential Cleaner, eventually he can take over responsibility for putting a winning team on the floor.

Few people can be exceptional at everything, so sometimes you have to experiment before you find the right result, a process that could have led to Michael's playing center in the NBA. Before the 1984 NBA draft, the Portland Trail Blazers called Bob Knight—who was coaching the USA Olympic basketball team that summer, which included Michael—and asked his opinion on whom they should take with the second pick in the draft. Everyone knew Houston would take Hakeem Olajuwon with the first pick, but no one (including Portland) was sure whether Portland would take Sam Bowie or Michael Jordan with the second pick.

"Take Jordan," said Knight.

"Right," said Portland, "but we need a center."

"Play him at center," Knight said.

Michael could probably have done it too. But most people don't have that option. You have to look at your teammates, your employees, and see what they *can* do, not what they *can't*. People who evaluate talent will always take the negative: "He can't do this, he can't do that." Okay, what *can* he do? He got this far for a reason, how did he get here? We've established what he can't do, so let's stop waiting for him to do it. Let's find out what he can do and put him in the system where he can succeed.

Everyone is given some ability at birth. Not everyone finds out what that ability is. Sometimes you find it on your own, sometimes it has to be shown to you. Either way, it's there. At the same time, there are abilities you are not given. Our challenge in life is to use the abilities we have, and to compensate for the abilities we don't have. It's completely instinctive; we compensate in order to survive. Individuals with limited vision frequently have heightened hearing; people with certain disabilities discover they have extraordinary talents in other areas. Something is given and something is taken away. I know countless athletes who are blessed with incredible physical gifts: height, skill, strength, speed . . . but no work ethic, or no support system, no way to use or develop or take advantage of those skills. Successful people compensate for what they don't have; unsuccessful people make excuses, blame everyone else, and never get past the deficiencies. A true leader can see past those deficiencies, identify the abilities, and get the most out of that individual.

A Cooler wonders what's going to happen.
A Closer watches things happen.
A Cleaner makes things happen.

I got deep into this discussion with a client during one of those "in case of emergency, break glass" meetings during the playoffs. The entire time we were together, we just talked. No physical stuff. Zero. Didn't stretch him before the game, didn't warm him up, didn't go to the gym. Just sat around and talked.

He was upset with some of his teammates, frustrated by what he believed they couldn't do. When you're so extraordinary at your craft, when your talent is so natural and your skill is so elevated, it's hard to understand that not everyone is like you and can do what you do. It's not a matter of their trying more or working harder, they really just can't do it. And if it's not handled right, it will destroy your entire team or office or wherever you have elite performers surrounded by less gifted colleagues.

We talked about every guy on the team, focusing on

all the players' strengths instead of their weaknesses. I told him that as the leader, his job was to recognize his players' talents and put them in situations where they could use those talents. Yes, we know this guy might mentally check out, and that guy isn't going to take a shot under pressure. We know this guy can deliver during the regular season, but in the playoffs he's going to look like the D League player he really is. So don't put the player in a position where it will matter. Work with the strengths, and everything else you get beyond that will be a bonus. You control this. Take charge of the situation and make it work in your favor.

"*But,*" I added, "you also have to recognize you're so competitive that you're crushing them with your disapproval. You don't realize the impact you have on everyone else because your wiring is completely different. When you're shaking your head or yelling at them, they shut down. And I know you love these guys, so they need to feel that you're backing them, not turning against them."

"I'm not doing that," he said.

Yes, you are. When you say something to an individual, and then you turn away before he can respond or make a comment back to you, you're making your point, and you're not letting him have his say. You have to see how someone reacts, so you know what's coming next. Is his head down? Is he angry? Are you motivating him or doing the opposite? When you hit someone with a negative attack, it doesn't energize him, it just brings him down. You're not going to win these guys over by making them feel worthless.

He got it. By the next game, he was literally meeting his teammates at half-court, patting them on the ass, showing his support . . . and if that's what it takes, that's what you have to do.

But for any leader, it's hard to resist the temptation to take over and just get things done. Kobe's job is to get 30–40 points per game. As soon as you tell him to start worrying about other players getting their points and feeling involved, you're pulling him out of his game. Obviously it's also his job to lead the team, but his main focus can't be on how many shots the other guys are taking. Let them worry about that, let them come up to your level. Remember, when a Cleaner gives you an opportunity, be ready, because he won't ask you again if you blow it. It's easier for him to just do the job himself, and if he's going down with the ship, he's going to make sure he's the captain.

A Cleaner's job is to take control and determine what has to happen to get results. You have a coach telling you this, players wanting that . . . but if you're the guy in the middle with the responsibility and the talent, all fingers are pointing at you, win or lose. Not just in sports, but in anything. When you're the guy they hired to make things happen, those things better happen or you won't be that guy for long. You are responsible. If there's going to be a mistake, you have to be the one to make it so you can turn it around immediately and get everyone back on track. It's all on you.

But as that guy, you also need to have everybody else, all the chemistry, going the same way with you. For every chief, there has to be a tribe, and at some point you have to let everyone in the tribe experience what it's like to be the chief so they can all see the intricacies and issues and texture of what happens at the top and recognize what's happening in the big picture rather than getting stuck in their own little scenes. And usually, as soon as you give them the entire view and tell them it's theirs to manage, every little detail and personality and weakness and strength, as soon as you give them that moment of complete power and control, most of them say, "Um, no thanks." Easier to stay where they're at, safe and comfortable.

No one knows that better than the coaches, who not only have to figure out the tribe but manage the chiefs as well. The good ones understand the dynamic: let your Cleaners do their thing. Those who can't give up that control eventually coach themselves out of a job. A Cleaner player needs a Cleaner coach because they'll understand and respect what each other has to do. Cleaners never sell each other out, they just let the other guy take care of business. Phil understood what he had to do with Michael: You respect my job and I'll respect yours. Run a couple of plays that I need you to run, and then have at it. Phil never sought relationships with his players, he just put them in situations where they could succeed, and he didn't try to make people do what they couldn't. He's not an X-and-O guy, he's all about total instinct and a gut feel for the game. He sees personalities and measures what they can do.

With Pat Riley, another Cleaner, it's all about the end result; that's why he's been so successful. You have to do it his way, and if you don't, he's going to make you do it his way. For a while, there was a lot of buzz that if Erik Spoelstra couldn't coach the Heat to a title, Riley would come down to the floor and take over the job himself. The players were so fearful of that, they figured they'd better get it done for Spoelstra, who was merely tough, as opposed to Riley, who is a competitive juggernaut. Easier to deal with the apprentice than the master.

Doug Collins is the best X-and-O guy I've ever known. He sees everything three plays ahead of everyone else, and no one else realizes what's coming. Then he puts everyone in strategic situations that appear to make no sense until the entire play unfolds, and suddenly everything materializes. His basketball mind is off the charts. But he sometimes forgets that not everyone can do that. Guys like Riley, the Van Gundys, and Tom Thibodeau in Chicago, they tell you how it is and expect you to do it their way, which can create friction with some of the big-money superstars who *don't* want to do it that way. You tell these guys they're having three-hour practices, two-hour shootarounds, and pretty soon the players start to mutiny. They hear about other teams having shorter practices, less work . . . now they're questioning why they have to work so hard. You can get away with that when players are younger, but a lot of the veterans and guys who have already won something don't want to deal with it. So you'd better be winning, or your players won't buy into your philosophy.

Mike Krzyzewski and I have a good relationship; we've spent a lot of time talking over the years. He's the best at bringing in players who he knows will work in his system—*I have this big stud here, that guy with the high basketball IQ over there, this guy with the jump shot*— and he pieces them together so it all works. They're not always the most gifted athletes, but he knows exactly what will work for his team, recognizes what they can do, and puts them in situations where they can shine. That's why he's been such a great coach for the Olympic teams; he puts people where they need to be, not just where they want to be (which is a frequent challenge when you're dealing with a dozen superstars). John Calipari goes the other way, he wants the best athletes out there so he doesn't have to mastermind anything. A different way of achieving the same result—winning—but relying more on the players' ability to excel without a lot of coaching or teaching.

But regardless of how you build that team—any team, in sports or business or any endeavor—no matter how you snap the pieces into place, you need that one guy who never needs a fire lit under him, who commands respect and fear and attention and demands that others bring the same excellence to their performance that he demands of himself. He doesn't have to be the most skilled or gifted guy on the team, but he establishes an example that everyone else can follow.

The only way you can light other people on fire is to be lit yourself, from the inside. Professional, cool, focused. If you had a bad night and you can't show up the next day ready to go, or you can't show up at all, that doesn't affect just you, it affects everyone around you. A professional doesn't let other people down just because of personal issues. If you need to show up, you show up. You might detest every individual in the room, but if your presence makes them all feel better, if it pulls the team together, if it results in better performances, then you've helped yourself to get one step closer to your own goal. That's how you get others to come up to your level: show them where it is, and set the example that allows them to get there.

#1. When You're a Cleaner . . .

. . . You make decisions, not suggestions; you know the answer while everyone else is still asking questions.

Three things you will never hear me talk about in a good way:

Inner drive.

Passion.

Whether the glass is half-full or half-empty.

You know what they all have in common?

They all translate into "I thought about it, and did nothing."

What the hell is "inner drive"? Inner drive is nothing

more than thought without action, internal wanderings that never hit the pavement to go anywhere. Completely worthless until those thoughts become external and convert to action. What good is the drive on the inside? Where are the results? People who preach inner drive are dreamers with a lot of ideas and a lot of talk, and zero production. They tell you everything they're going to do, and then they do nothing. That's inner drive.

Let's move on.

Passion: a strong feeling or emotion for something or someone. Very nice. Now what? Are you just feeling it, or are you going to do something about it? I love hearing motivational speakers tell people to "follow your passion." Follow it? How about *work* at it. *Excel* at it. *Demand to be the best* at it. Follow it? Eh.

But my favorite: the timeless debate over whether some invisible glass is half-full or half-empty.

This is a concept invented by someone suffering from the complete inability to make decisions. Half-full or half-empty? You have something in the glass or you don't. If you like what's there, add more. If you don't, pour it out and start over. Otherwise, you're just staring at this nonexistent glass thinking, "Damn, there's no way to decide."

Bullshit. Of course there's a way to decide, you just don't want to commit to a decision. As soon as someone starts with the half-full/half-empty analysis, you know you're in for a long debate about nothing, with someone who can't or won't make a choice. To me it's the equivalent of a guy standing in the middle of a busy intersection crying, "I don't know!" while everyone around him screams, "Get out of the street!"

Trust yourself. Decide.

Every minute, every hour, every day that you sit around trying to figure out what to do, someone else is already doing it.

While you're trying to choose whether to go left or right, this way or that way, someone else is already there.

While you're paralyzed from overthinking and over-analyzing your next move, someone else went with his gut and beat you to it.

Make a choice, or a choice will be made for you.

Most people don't want to make decisions. They make suggestions, and they wait to see what everyone else thinks, so they can say, "It was just a suggestion." They know the right answer, but can't act because if something goes wrong, they'll have to take responsibility and then they can't blame anyone else. Meanwhile, someone else is going to make a decision, and when it works, he's getting all the credit. And maybe the choice he made isn't one that works for anyone but him, but since no one else took charge, too bad for everyone else.

A Cleaner makes decisions because there's no chance in the world he's going to let anyone else make a decision for him. He may ask your opinion and add it to every-thing else he knows, but he's not going to do what anyone else tells him; he's still going to follow his own instincts. And once he decides, it's set in stone; he doesn't care what anyone else thinks of his choice, and he's going to live with the outcome.

He decides, and then he acts.

I'll give credit to the Coolers for this: they have the flexibility and willingness to rethink their decisions and change directions if you give them a reason. A Cleaner will just tell you to fuck off.

You can waste a lifetime sitting around overthinking possible ways to look at something. On one hand . . . but on the other hand . . . but then on this hand . . . Stop it, you only have two hands, and that's already too many.

One guy is telling you, "Think positive!" while someone else is saying, "I don't mean to be negative, but . . ." I don't believe in thinking positive *or* thinking negative. Plenty of "experts" have made a lot of money taking a stand on this; good for them, but keep them away from my players. The positive thinkers want you to only visualize your success; the negative thinkers want you to focus on everything that could go wrong. Well, visualizing anything doesn't make it a reality, and overthinking imaginary problems just generates fear and anxiety. I want you armed with reflexes and instinct, not Xanax.

You'll never hear me say, "We have a problem." We might have a situation that needs to be addressed, or an issue we have to resolve, but never a problem. Why automatically cast something as a negative? Instincts don't recognize positive or negative. There's only a situation, your response, and an outcome. If you're ready for anything, you're not thinking about whether it's a good situation or a bad situation, you're looking at the whole picture. And if you *are* thinking about it, you're out of the Zone, distracted and wasting energy and emotion instead of focusing only on what you have to do. Thinking doesn't achieve outcomes, only action does. Prepare yourself with everything you'll need to succeed, then act. You don't need a hundred people to back you up and be your safety net. Your preparation and your instincts are your safety net.

You suddenly get a great idea, something completely comes alive in your mind, you mention it to a couple people . . . and they stare at you blankly. Suddenly you lose all your enthusiasm. Why? It's still the same idea you loved a few hours ago. What happened?

Stop thinking.

After that first initial thought, that first instantaneous gut reaction, why give in to the weakness of second-guessing and doubt and analysis that inevitably follow? Are you listening to others, or to your own instincts? Are you taking advice from people who know what they're talking about, or those who only see failure? As soon as you allow yourself to start overthinking your decisions, you start saying things like "I'll sleep on it" or "Let's put it on the back burner" or any one of the stupid clichés that mean "I don't trust myself to make a decision." Back burner? The back burner is for cooling things. You've just cooled a hot idea. And then you'll forget about it altogether and quit, never knowing how close you might have been to success.

Speaking of clichés, here's another tribute to indecision and apathy:

Good things come to those who wait.

No, good things come to those who *work*. I understand the value of not rushing into things—you want to be quick, not careless—but you still have to work toward a result, not just sit back and wait for something to happen. You can't wait. The decision you don't make on Monday will still be waiting for you on Tuesday, and by then two new decisions will have to be dealt with, and if you still don't make those decisions, you'll have three more on Wednesday. Pretty soon, you're so overwhelmed by everything you still haven't dealt with that you become completely paralyzed and can't do anything.

Meanwhile, as you sit back doing nothing because you're afraid to make a mistake, someone else is out there making all kinds of mistakes, learning from them, and getting to where you wanted to be. And probably laughing at your weakness.

And when you do finally force yourself to make a decision, what do you choose? Almost always, you go back to your first reaction, the first thing you thought of when the whole process began. You already knew. Why didn't you just trust yourself the first time?

You can't rely on others to jump up and make your dreams happen. They have their own dreams, they're not worrying about yours. People might be willing to help if they can, but ultimately, it's on you. Get the best people around you, know your strengths and weaknesses, and trust others to do what they do best. But in the end, it's still your responsibility. Make a plan, and execute.

What's your plan? Everything starts with a simple thought. Every idea, every invention, every plan, every creation . . . it started with a thought. But to bring the thought to life, you have to put a plan together. Starting a workout, training for a sport, launching a business . . . you can just think about it, or you can create the plan that will get you there. Be realistic: How much time do you have? How much time will you commit? Is it going to be a priority in your schedule, or are you going to fit it in around your other commitments? Make a plan that truly reflects your goals and interests, and you'll be more likely to execute. Why pretend you're going to work out every single day when you know you're only going to do it three times a week?

You make a choice and stand by it.

Most people can't do that. They're content to "wing it" or "see what happens." Come on, you already know what's going to happen if you go into it that way— whatever you started is going to fall apart. But that's what most people do, they "test the waters" before jumping in. Why? Unless you suspect those waters are churning with crocodiles, what's the worst thing that can happen if you take the plunge? You get wet. A Cleaner thinks, "No problem, I'll swim." Most people just stand at the edge shivering and looking for a towel.

Oh, you can't swim? Fine, then tell me what you *can* do. Why stand at the water's edge feeling sorry for yourself? Go a different way, excel in another area, while everyone else is just competing for space in the same pool. You don't become unstoppable by following the crowd, you get there by doing something better than anyone else can do it, and proving every day why you're the best at what you do.

You must know someone like this: He can do everything. This week he's a blogger and a songwriter and a motivator, last week he was teaching tennis two nights a week and working as a sushi chef. And on the weekends he's rebuilding a 1955 Maserati. You listen to him and feel as if you've never done a thing in your life. Until you listen more closely and discover that like a lot of people, this is someone dabbling in a lot of things and succeeding at none. I listen to those people and think, "As far as I can tell, the only thing you're good at is keeping busy."

I want to hear someone say, "I do *this.*" Ask Kobe what he does, and he says, "I give out numbers." Numbers? "Yep, I gave them eighty-one, I gave them a triple double, I gave those guys sixty-one. . . ." People love to comment on how he doesn't pass enough, but his job is to score points and give out those numbers, and that's what he does.

I'll tell a player, "In order for you to reach your highest ability, this is going to be your number one focus. I want to make you excellent at this one thing. You can be average and above average at the other things, but when people talk about someone who can do this, you're going to be the first name on the list."

Otherwise, most people want to show they can do everything, which ultimately detracts from their real abilities. If you're not a 3-point shooter, don't take those shots. If you're not a home-run hitter, if you're the guy who's supposed to get on base and steal, do that. People get paid a fortune for being the expert at one thing, so that anytime others need that one thing done, you're the only one they're calling.

Years ago, I went with Michael to an FBI training facility where there's a practice range for the most elite sharpshooters in the world. There's one guy out there alone, practicing his craft, over and over. The target is four hundred yards away—four football fields. He has to get in his truck, drive to the target, set it up, and drive back to where we're standing. He gets his gun with the scope, takes aim, one shot—*foom*—we didn't even hear it go. Then we get in the truck with him and drive back to the target. Hit it dead fucking center. We would have been impressed if he'd hit the target anywhere. Four hundred yards. Dead center.

Michael asked him how many people use that target range. He said, "Just me." So unless he had visitors like us, which didn't happen too often, he was alone working on this one shot, over and over, so when people in the military need someone who can hit that kind of target, they call him. No one knows what this guy does every day to be this good. People just know he can deliver results.

Figure out what you do, then do it. And do it better than anyone else.

And then let everything else you do build around that; stay with what you know. Being great at one thing doesn't mean you can also run a restaurant or a car dealership or a line of sportswear. Bill Gates is not going to launch a line of sportswear. Most likely, neither should you.

No matter how many years I'm in this business, I still shake my head at pro athletes who can't make the decision to commit themselves to excellence. This is your body, your livelihood, you only get a few years to ride this wave. Are you going to ride it or lie on the beach whining that the water's too cold?

One of the hardest decisions for an athlete is to determine how much fatigue and pain he can endure, and how far he can push himself. Everyone plays with pain, there's always something going on physically. The question is, how do you keep that from affecting you mentally? If you know you're going to have constant pain, can you get comfortable being uncomfortable?

When some guys get injured and the doctor tells them they can't work out, they're fine with that, it's a relief and they don't miss it. When a Cleaner gets injured, he's going to find a way to work out or go crazy trying. You have to make a choice. You can listen to the doctor and have a safer, longer recovery, or you can take the shorter route, a quick fix, maybe not long-term quality but you'll be able to play. Depends how badly you want it.

If a Cleaner was put in a situation where he had to remove a body part to survive, he wouldn't think twice about it. He'd figure out a way to adapt without it. Eh, it's a finger, I can go without it. Lose a finger or lose a season? He's losing the finger.

Kobe has a finger that moves in all kinds of ways a finger isn't supposed to move. A normal person would have it surgically repaired. But what's the advantage to him, other than he won't be able to bend his finger all the way over backward? The surgery will cost him nine months of basketball. Is that worth it?

Cleaners have a high tolerance for physical and mental pain; it's another great challenge to see how much they can take, what they can endure, how well they can play when they're not healthy. Michael's legendary flu game during the 1997 NBA Finals . . . Kobe's famed flu game during the 2012 season. You have to beware of a Cleaner when he's physically sick because his body has totally challenged him to see what he's capable of. And because he's not as physically strong, he'll find another way to beat you, usually by turning up his mental game. Sickness, physical or mental, is one of the best ways to put a person in the Zone: his survival instincts kick in and give him an extra gear for fighting back from a weakened state.

About Michael's famous flu: I think most people recognize by now that he probably didn't actually have the flu that night in Utah; more likely it was food poisoning. Shortly before becoming ill, he had ordered in a late-night dinner from the only place we could find open in Park City, and when six guys showed up to deliver it, I felt something was wrong. Soon after, he was curled up on the floor, miserable and shaking and sicker than I had ever seen him. Yet he had the grit and determination to play the next night, scoring 38 in what would become one of the defining games of his entire career. "Probably the most difficult thing I've ever done," he said later.

Amazing what someone can do when everything is on the line.

• • •

Some decisions can be life-altering: Should you retire? Have the surgery? Give up your dream?

Some decisions are less challenging.

After every game, I used to ask Michael one question: Five, six, or seven?

As in, what time are we hitting the gym tomorrow morning?

And he'd snap back a time, and that was it. Especially after a loss, when there wasn't a whole lot else to say. No discussion, no debate, no lame attempt to convince me he needed the morning off. You good? I'm good. See you in the morning.

And the next morning at whatever time he'd decided, he'd awaken to find me standing outside his door. No matter what had happened the night before—good game, bad game, soreness, fatigue—he was up working out every morning while most of the other guys slept.

Interesting how the guy with the most talent and success spent more time working out than anyone else.

Kobe is the same; he's insatiable in his desire to work. Some days we'll go back to the gym twice a day and once more at night, trying different things, working on certain issues, always looking for that extra edge. At his level of excellence, there's no room for error, and no one—*no one*—in the game today works harder or invests more in his body and surrounds himself with the right people to keep it in peak condition.

But it's still not easy, and Kobe makes that decision, every day, to do the work. Again: the most talented guy working harder than anyone else.

It's a choice.

Each of Kobe's workouts takes around ninety minutes, and a half hour of that is spent just working on his wrists, fingers, ankles . . . all the details.

That's how the best get better—they sweat the details.

And every workout, at some point he'll glare at me and ask, What we got left? Because let's face it, the work is hard and tedious, and sometimes that hoop looks as if it's a thousand feet in the air and you're trying to reach it wearing lead boots.

But he does the work because if he can't put that ball in the hoop, everything else goes away. That's a choice.

It all comes back to this, no matter what you do in life: Are you willing to make the decision to succeed? Are you going to stand by that decision or quit when it gets hard? Will you choose to keep working when everyone else tells you to quit? Pain comes in all sorts of disguises—physical, mental, emotional. Do you need to be pain-free? Or can you push past it and stand by your commitment and decision to go further? It's your choice. The outcome is on you.

#1. WHEN YOU'RE
A CLEANER . . .

. . . You don't have to love the work, but you're addicted to the results.

A Cooler makes you wish you paid him less.
A Closer asks how much and then decides how hard he'll work.
A Cleaner doesn't think about the money; he just does the work
and knows you'll be grateful for the privilege of paying him.

Finally, the big day. Perfect knot in your $200 tie, Mom has a new dress, the whole family is by your side. Someone suddenly whispers in your ear—this is it. The commissioner is at the podium. "With the eleventh pick . . ." You don't hear anything else. The first person to hug you is your agent.

Congratulations, today is the beginning of the end of your career.

Did you exhale? Did you think, "I'm finally here, set for life"? Or did you think, "I have a lot of work to do"?

Most guys, on the day they're drafted, go out to celebrate. Kobe went to the gym to practice.

Making it to the top is not the same as making it at the top. True for any business; getting the job doesn't mean you're keeping the job; winning the client doesn't mean he's staying forever. Most people seem to understand that. They get a big opportunity and usually realize they now have to go out and earn that salary, working even harder to prove they deserve it.

But if you're an athlete who just got rich quick, the day you sign that contract can easily be the beginning of the end. You're already on the pedestal. Your shoe deal is in place. Now you're not just known by the team you play for, you're known by your brand affiliation. Instead of spending the summer working on your game, you're traveling the world pitching your sportswear. Your group of "friends" just grew ten times larger than it was a week ago. And you're no longer dreaming about what you can do for the game, but what the game can do for you.

You took what was handed to you, and that was the end.

I'm using athletes as an example here, but you know it applies to anyone else as well: What have you been handed and what are you willing to earn?

At some point, you got a gift: maybe you were blessed with talent, or you inherited the family business, or someone took a chance on you and let you in the door. Then what? Doors swing two ways. Did you shut it on the competition or on yourself?

There's nothing wrong with receiving a gift; that's where the challenge begins. Like a lot of people with a crazy dream, I saw an opportunity, worked hard to develop it, and never stopped working to see how far I could take it. Whenever other people in my business want to rip me, they say, "Sure, the guy started with Michael Jordan, it's not hard to train the best." If you think it's "not hard" to take the best and find ways to make him better, you've never had to face that challenge. It's easy to improve on mediocrity, not so easy to improve on excellence.

Cleaner Law: when you reduce your competition to whining that you "got lucky," you know you're doing something right.

There are no shortcuts, and there is no luck. People always say "good luck" in a pressure situation. No. It's not about luck, I don't believe in luck. There are facts and opportunities and realities, and how you respond to them determines whether you succeed or fail. Even the lottery isn't about luck: there's a set of numbers, either you get them right or you don't. When the game is on the line, you don't want to hear "good luck"; it suggests you're not prepared. When you're headed to a job interview, you don't need luck. You need to know you're prepared and in control, and you're not relying on some random events or mystical intervention. Luck becomes a convenient excuse when things don't go your way, and a rationale for staying comfortable while you wait for luck to determine your fate. You can't be relentless if you're willing to gamble everything on the unknown.

It doesn't matter what you get handed, it's what you do after you receive it that affords you the privilege of saying, "I did this on my own." If you get that gift and decide you're all set, you stand no chance—zero—of ever understanding greatness or excellence. Now you're the opposite of unstoppable. You stopped all on your own.

Dwyane is the perfect example of receiving nothing but talent, and taking it to the top. From a small high school in Chicago not known for its great basketball program, he was barely recruited by any colleges and ended up at Marquette. He didn't even play his freshman year because of academic reasons. But he knew what it was going to take if he had any chance of making it to the pros, and he fought his way back. In 2003 he was drafted by the Miami Heat, the fifth pick after LeBron James, Darko Milicic, Carmelo Anthony, and Chris Bosh.

That's right, of the Big Three, Dwyane Wade was the last one drafted.

He arrived in Miami without billboards, megamillion-dollar shoe deals, or a crown. He just showed up and played. Three years later, he had his first championship ring. It would be years before anyone drafted ahead of him would do the same.

You cannot understand what it means to be relentless until you have struggled to possess something that's just out of your reach. Over and over, as soon as you touch it, it moves farther away. But something inside you—that killer instinct—makes you keep going, reaching, until you finally grab it and fight with all your might to keep holding on. Anyone can take what's sitting right in front of him. Only when you're truly relentless can you understand the determination to keep pursuing a target that never stops moving.

No question, those who are gifted get to the top faster than anyone else. So what? Is that your excuse for not reaching as high? The challenge is staying there, and most people don't have the balls to put in the work. If you want to be elite, you have to earn it. Every day, everything you do. Earn it. Prove it. Sacrifice.

No shortcuts. You can't fight the elephants until you've wrestled the pigs, messed around in the mud, handled the scrappy, dirty issues that clutter everyday life, so you can be ready for the heavy stuff later. There's no way you can be prepared to compete and survive at anything if you start with the elephants; no matter how good your instincts are, you'll always lack the basic knowledge needed to build your arsenal of attack weapons. And when you're surrounded by those elephants, they'll know they're looking at a desperate newcomer.

One summer I had about fifty guys in the gym, a combination of veterans and predraft players, including one young man who had never spent a single day wrestling a pig. He had gone to good schools with the top coaches and came from a great family that made sure he had whatever he needed. He worked hard, but everything had been too easy, from scholarships to trophies, and he became a big star without paying a whole lot of dues. He expected to be drafted high and had no idea how things worked in the real world, unprotected by the college environment and supportive followers.

He was a marked man from the minute he touched the ball. Every single player in the gym that day had one mission: fuck this kid up. Not nice, but competition rarely is. And because he had never been exposed to that level of heat and anger, he completely crumbled. He couldn't do a thing—out of those fifty guys in the gym that day, he ranked fifty-first—and he learned the hard way that there's not a magazine cover or a parade that can help you when you're not prepared.

People who start at the top never understand what they missed at the bottom. The guy who started by sorting the mail, or cleaning the restaurant late at night, or fixing the equipment at the gym, that's the guy who knows how things get done. After he's eventually worked his way up through the ranks, he knows how everything works, why it works, what to do when it stops working. That's the guy who will have longevity and value and impact, because he knows what it took to get to the top. You can't claim you ran a marathon if you started at the seventeenth mile.

Most people are looking for an elevator instead of taking the stairs—they want the easy route. People quit their workouts and diets because they're too hard. They stop advancing in their careers and lives because it's too much work. Guys make it to the pros and then don't want to play for coaches who are too tough. They can't deal with being uncomfortable so they seek the shortcut, and when they can't find it, they quit.

For all of Michael's amazing moves and unforgettable moments, he knew none of that could happen without the fundamentals. Those basic moves he had practiced over and over and over since he was a kid made everything else possible. He didn't work on being flashy, he worked on being consistent, and he worked on it relentlessly. Cleaners don't care about instant gratification; they invest in the long-term payoff.

Ask yourself honestly, what would you have to sacrifice to have what you really want? Your social life? Relationships? Credit cards? Free time? Sleep? Now answer this question: What are you *willing* to sacrifice? If those two lists don't match up, you don't want it badly enough.

No matter what you do, if you're in it for the money or the attention, if you're not willing to put in the hard work and the commitment, if you're okay with just being okay, I have to ask you, why?

Look, it's enough for a lot of people, I'm not judging. They don't want the pressure and stress, they don't want to sacrifice time with friends and family, they want to party when the mood strikes, sleep late when they can, and get up and go to bed with limited worries and responsibilities and pressure. I get that. It's a much easier way to experience life.

But usually, those are the same people who look around at others who have more success and say, "I can't believe how lucky that guy is, I could do that if . . ." Stop. You could do that if . . . what? If you put in more time and effort? If you commit to whatever is making it work for him? If you're willing to pay the price he's paying? What's he doing that you can't do?

That's what I thought. You could do the same, and so much more. What's stopping you?

And even if you can't do it his way—and why should you?—why aren't you doing it your own way?

Don't be jealous of someone if you had the same opportunity and you let it slip away.

When did hard work become a skill? It doesn't take talent to work hard, anyone can do it. Show up, work hard, and listen. It takes a willingness to be dedicated, to improve, to be better. I don't care if you're a superstar or the weakest guy on the team, anyone can show up, work hard, and listen. Are you looking for that nonexistent shortcut, or are you ready to do things the right way? Do you want it easy, or do you want it great?

During the 2011–12 NBA season, which started two months late due to a labor dispute, a lot of players suffered serious injuries. Almost all the blame was placed squarely on the lockout, the shortened season, too many games with too little rest. When the labor standoff ended, and the league rushed into action with limited workouts and practice, everyone complained that the players had no time to get ready. The consequences were immediately obvious: many players were out of shape, poorly conditioned, unprepared to play, and on their way to being injured, some for days or weeks, others for the entire season.

But here's my question: Why were the players out of shape, poorly conditioned, and unprepared to play?

Seriously, all those months, sitting around waiting for the lockout to end . . . what else did they have to do?

When you use your body for a living, you have one job and it requires one thing: work hard to stay in peak condition. That's it. Protect your body and your skills, get in shape and stay that way. It's a year-round commitment, not a hobby. You're supposed to be the best in the world, you're one of only a few hundred athletes who get to have this job, and you can't work out because you don't know when the season is starting? Who the hell cares when the season is starting? Get your ass in the gym!

Yet when it was clear that the NBA season would start late, or perhaps not at all, the majority of players trained less (or not at all), deciding they could put in the hard work when necessary. I heard it over and over: didn't want to pay for trainers, didn't want to waste the time and effort required to get to that level of preparedness. Great, now we've got some of the greatest athletes on earth putting in the same effort as the average guy at the health club. Maybe less. "If we had known when the season was going to start . . ." Stop it. What difference did it make? You should have been ready to go, instead of planning to do the "real" work when the season was ready to roll. You can't prepare for the intensity of an entire NBA season at the last minute, especially one that would be condensed and allow little time for rest and recovery. Oh, you didn't know the schedule was going to be condensed? So what? You should still have been ready.

One guy who took no shortcuts getting ready for the season was Kobe. Given his history of injuries and his long list of accomplishments, it would have been easy for him to take the summer off, get some rest, and wait for the league to settle its issues. Instead, he invested the time working out, training, and preparing to be better than ever. So when most players were relaxing with light workouts that did nothing to prepare them for the grueling months ahead, Kobe and I were in a gym most of the summer and fall, putting in hours every day, usually twice a day and sometimes more.

When the season finally started on Christmas Day, when other players were still trying to find their legs and their shot, he was already mentally and physically ready. In the months that followed, he played through (a) knee pain, (b) torn wrist ligaments, (c) a broken nose, and (d) a concussion, and he did not miss a single game until he was kicked in the shin playing against the Hornets in April, an injury that sidelined him for seven games and forced him to take an unwanted rest that ultimately cost him the scoring title. Until that injury, he never asked to sit out, never took a shortcut. No one but Kobe can know the pain and discomfort he endured, but the hard work he had already put in paid off, and his body allowed him to keep going when most athletes would have had to sit.

In anything you do, it takes no talent to work hard. You just have to want to do it. I could tell you so many stories about athletes blessed with incredible physical talent—size, power, pure athletic excellence—who end up playing sports only because that's where their gifts direct them. They don't love it or even like it, but that's where they end up because they're so physically extraordinary. So they have no motivation to do more because they don't crave the end result. They're happy to be there if there's a parade at the end, but if there's not, they're okay with that too.

You can tell those players, "For the same money you can go to this team but you'll probably sit on the bench, or you can go to this other team and play every day, but first they need you to drop forty pounds and get in shape," and every time they'll say, "I'm getting paid either way? Fuck it, I don't need to get in shape."

I had a player who fit so well where he was, they loved him there, and when his contract was up, they offered him $42 million, which was probably $32 million more than he was worth. Then another team offered him $48 million. Please, I said, stay where you are. You don't fit with the other team, they won't know how to use you, it's a mistake. Of course he took the money and changed teams. And that extra $6 million has probably cost him at least $20 million because—surprise—it didn't work out and he cheated himself out of what could have been a longer and more successful career.

Spend your career on the bench for the right team and you can walk away with a nice bonus and a ring. Good enough, if good enough is what you set out to achieve. You made some money sitting down. But money doesn't make you smart, it doesn't make you a good businessman, and it sure doesn't make you better looking. Most of the time it makes you soft, complacent, and mistakenly confident about your future. But you may not realize any of that for a long time, because as soon as people see those dollar signs, you're suddenly going to be more powerful than you ever imagined.

Until the money runs out, the party ends, they all move on to the next guy, and you can't get anyone to return your texts.

When everything you do is about the money, if that's the end result you crave, what happens when it ends? Because it's going to end, whether you want to admit it or not. Someone else is going to make more, do more, and be more because you did nothing but sit back and say, "Look at me, I'm rich."

Anyone can start something. Few can finish. Priorities change if you don't constantly protect and defend them. You stop caring about keeping up with the competition, unless you mean the competition to have more stuff than the next guy, and instead of being addicted to building your career and your legacy, you become addicted to building bigger houses and more garages and adding more names to the party list. And pretty soon, you're just part of a long list of nobodies with declining talent who bumbled themselves out of a job.

Part of the commitment to hard work is knowing what you have to give up to do the work . . . learning to control whatever pulls you away from your mission. You start having a little success, people notice you, it feels good . . . and maybe you start feeling a little satisfied and privileged. Trust me: privilege is a poison unless you know how to manage it.

Anywhere you go, no matter what you do, there are going to be distractions. What are you willing to give up? Every year by Labor Day, Michael would shut down everything outside of basketball and just train. Three workouts a day: workout, golf break, workout, lunch, golf break, workout, dinner, bed. Every day. No commercial shoots, no promotional tours, no events. Just work, because he knew better than anyone else that all the outside stuff was the result of hard work on the inside, not the other way around. Shoe deals and commercials don't make you an icon. Being unstoppable makes you an icon. And being unstoppable only comes with hard work.

Take care of business. When your career is over, if you want to weigh four hundred pounds and lie in bed eating potato chips all day, I don't care. But for now, your body is your tool, that's what's allowing you to do your job and get a contract and pay all these bills.

I'm going to show up ready to work every day, and I expect the same of you. So tell me the night before if you're going out, if you're not going to be worth anything the next day, so I know how to make my adjustments. I need to know if there's something wrong with your game, or if you got overserved and can't see straight. Maybe we'll go a little easy on this day, but we'll make it up here and there. The more you communicate with me, the better results I can get for you. But just the truth, and keep it simple. "I feel like garbage today." Fine. Heard you. I don't want the explanation. If I need more, I will ask you. If I think you're seriously fucking up, I will tell you. Otherwise, show me you care about your career and I'll care as well.

Be professional. That's the one thing I admired so much about Michael when he was going through the grief of his father's death; he came back and did what he had to do, at an even higher level. Dwyane, going through an ugly divorce and uglier custody battle, still showed up every day like the professional he is. Cleaner Law: When you're going through a world of pain, you never hide. You show up to work ready to go, you face adversity and your critics and those who judge you, you step into the Zone and perform at that top level when everyone is expecting you to falter. That's being a professional.

Neglecting your body and your skill . . . not professional. Every year I'll talk to a frustrated GM or agent about some young player who's trashing his entire future because he can't get this right. Instead of investing time and resources refining his skills and improving his conditioning so he can make it in the league, he's telling everyone it's too expensive and exhausting to train all summer and he needs the off-season to relax. He's driving a $150,000 car, wearing a ten-pound diamond watch and a gold chain around his neck like a boa constrictor, and he won't spend ten grand to guarantee he continues to make $10 million? Sorry, there's no off-season when you're serious about being a winner. But, hey, you can enjoy that off-season permanently when you're cut by the team.

Do the work. There is no privilege greater than the pressure to excel, and no greater reward than earning the respect and fear of others who can only stand in awe of your results.

#1. When You're a Cleaner . . .

. . . You'd rather be feared than liked.

A Cooler keeps his opinions to himself.
A Closer will say what he thinks, but only behind your back.
A Cleaner will tell you straight to your face what he thinks, whether you like it or not.

I'm always intrigued by the interaction between rival players, particularly when jealousy and competitive bitterness show themselves on the floor. As someone who has watched hundreds of thousands of hours of basketball, I know I'm not imagining it when players get frozen out in an All-Star Game or in the Olympics, as other players conspire to keep the ball away from them, in open defiance of the game plan and the coach.

We're not talking about Cleaners here; a Cleaner wants to beat you when you're at your best, not when you're standing there without the ball. A "freeze-out" is the kind of petty bullshit you typically see from younger players who start feeling a little proud of themselves, and decide to show the chief that the tribe is taking over.

In a way, it's sort of amusing because, let's face it, if you're going to grab some spotlight and show off, it seems silly to do it in All-Star and Olympic Games, where the competition is questionable at best. If that's the best way you can get the oohs and aahs, do what you have to do.

But heaven help you if you choose to freeze out a true Cleaner; he sees what you're doing, and he'll never forget. Because when you're the best of the best, someone is always going to try to catch you, and you love watching them try.

A Cooler is liked.

A Closer is respected.

A Cleaner is feared, and then respected for doing exactly what everyone feared he'd do.

A Cleaner moves silently under the surface—he makes no waves, so you never know what he's doing. You can't see him or hear him. You may not even know who he is. But when he's ready for you to find out, he does it with a tsunami that comes with no warning. You have no idea what's coming until you've been completely rocked, and by then it's too late for you to do anything but be swept away.

He will make no effort to get you to like him; he doesn't care. But he'll do everything possible—and succeed—to make sure you fear him.

How does it feel when you don't know what's about to happen? You get nervous, distracted . . . you're looking over your shoulder, wondering and worrying. If I want to get into another guy's head, I'll whisper in someone else's ear while he's watching. I may just be whispering about where we should go to dinner after the game, but now the first guy is wondering what we're saying instead of focusing on what he's supposed to be doing. Knocks him right out of his Zone.

Do you want to be the guy worrying, or the guy quietly making everyone else worry?

This is what makes Kobe one of the greats of all time: He doesn't tell you what he's thinking or what he's going to do. He just does it. He makes others fear his next move and respect his ability to execute it.

When Dwyane broke Kobe's nose and gave him the concussion during the All-Star Game, and Kobe wanted to see him face-to-face before he'd go to the hospital, it wasn't about vengeance or retaliation or settling the score. It was about the law and order of the jungle, two animals instinctively facing off, the lion king getting up on that rock so the rest of the jungle could see who was in charge. One direct, silent look that says, "I still own this, motherfucker."

Fear and respect: let them know you were there by

your actions, not your words or emotions. You don't have to be loud to be the focus of attention. Think of the Godfather, world-class Cleaner and the quietest guy in the room, surrounded by everyone else waiting to see what he would do or say, and he never had to say a word to get his message across.

Or the parent who just gives the kids that look; no lecture, no speeches. One look, maybe a word or two, and there's nothing more to say. Complete control. That's fear and respect in action.

The loudest guy in the room is the one with the most to prove, and no way to prove it. A Cleaner has no need to announce his presence; you'll know he's there by the way he carries himself, always cool and confident. He's never the blowhard telling you how great he is; he's the quiet guy focused on results, because results are all that matter. A thief doesn't walk into a crowded store screaming, "I'm stealing!" He comes in quietly, subtly executing his plan before anyone notices. And he's long gone by the time you notice your watch is missing.

When people start broadcasting what they're going to do, and how great they're going to be when they do it, it's a sure sign they're still trying to convince themselves. If you already know, you don't have to talk about it. Talk never goes up in price, it's always free, and you usually get what you pay for.

The Olympics are a classic example of this. I've been to the Olympics with several of the USA basketball teams since the 1992 Dream Team games in Barcelona, and in any sport you can see the difference between the athletes who are already thinking about fame and endorsements, and those who understand you have to *win* something first. The networks and Olympic sponsors are promoting them even before they arrive at the games, they're completely drenched in hype. Moms, dads, coaches, trainers, nutritionists . . . everyone wants a share of the spotlight.

And there's always at least one athlete who can't resist: He talks about whom he's going to beat, how he's going to beat them, how he trained to get there, and then . . . splat. He can't measure up to the talk. His focus drains into the cameras, not into his performance.

I'm sure most people respect swimmer Michael Phelps for all the medals. I respect him more for his ability to let those medals do the talking. While other swimmers were promising to knock him off the podium and take all the gold, he said nothing in response, never showed what he was thinking. When he got off to a slow start, and people started to wonder if he was "done," he pulled even farther back into himself, remembered why he was there, and crushed the rest of the events.

That's how you intimidate your opponents without saying a single word.

Michael Jordan had the best intimidation technique I've ever seen. You can't do this anymore, but before certain playoff games, he'd walk into the opponents' locker room on the pretense he had a pal on the other side and he had to say hello. Now, if you really knew him, you knew that was completely ridiculous because Michael didn't care about saying hello to anyone, especially before a game. But try telling that to the guys in the other locker room, getting ready to play. The whole team would be sitting there, thinking about facing the world champion Chicago Bulls . . . and in walks Michael Jordan. I don't care how long any of them had been in the game, when Michael Jordan walked in, you'd notice. He'd open that door, and the whole place would suddenly go completely silent. Everyone and everything just stopped. You could see every pair of eyes following him, watching, wondering, waiting to see what he was going to do. He'd only stay a minute, just long enough for a brief handshake with whomever he knew (or pretended to know), a quick nod around the room, and he'd leave as quickly as he'd arrived.

The Black Cat, we called him. There and gone before you knew what had happened.

He wouldn't give it another thought. But for the stunned players sitting in that locker room, they could think of nothing else. Mission accomplished: He'd gone into their space and lodged himself in their heads for the entire game. Now they're no longer thinking about what they have to do, they're thinking about him. Instead of clearing their minds and getting to that cool, focused performance Zone, their minds are heating up over #23. He's got the entire other team talking to each other about how many points the great Michael Jordan will score that night, how many he'd scored the night before, the suit he was wearing, the automobile he drove. They were no longer his opponents, they were just a bunch of fans in awe.

A player might score 20 points the night before facing the Bulls, then 2 points when he got to Chicago. And then 20 again in the next game against someone else. That wasn't strictly about the Bulls' defense; a guy's skill doesn't deteriorate for one game. What changed? Only his frame of mind. He was thinking about playing against Michael Jordan.

Wherever Michael went, there was that undeniable element of fear and respect. Everyone felt it. Every game, he'd do something unforgettable, and no one would know what it was going to be. Even he didn't always know what it was going to be. But he'd make you wait and wonder. He always gave the other team and the crowd a *wow* moment, sometimes an entire *wow* game. In the later years of his career, when he wasn't going to dunk every night, he'd still sneak one in every now and then just to let everyone know he could still do it. Not because he had to, but because he wanted to remind the rest of the league, "You're next." Even when he went to the Wizards, and everyone said he was done, he'd still find a way to stab you in the heart. *Just because I don't, doesn't mean I can't.*

Cleaners always leave behind a taste of the fear factor to give their next victims something to think about, so everyone knows they're coming; that's the undeniable edge they give themselves. That was one of Tiger's greatest weapons, knowing the rest of the field was looking back to see what he was doing, waiting for him to make his move. Every tournament, every round, every hole were all about him; the only thing anyone—including the competition—wanted to know was "What did Tiger do?" But when he was struck down by scandal and injury and his game deteriorated, the competition stopped worrying about him. He no longer commanded the fear and respect that had made him an unstoppable force. Everyone else's skills didn't just suddenly improve. But their mental focus did.

Athletes spend so much time working on their physical excellence they sometimes forget that respect isn't just about what you can do physically; you have to be able to perform intellectually and mentally as well. The way you conduct yourself in all areas of your life, your ability to show intelligence and class and self-control . . . those are the things that separate you from the rest of the pack.

Mental edge is everything in my line of work. If I have an altercation with a player, I don't stand a chance of beating him physically; I'm under six feet and possibly twice his age. But the result is going to be so much worse for him because I'm going to deal with him mentally. I don't work out like these guys do, I don't have to. They don't need me to be on their level physically, they need me to exceed their level mentally. I hear from young trainers all the time; they tell me about all their athletic achievements and how many years they've been working out. Great, you're physically fit, congratulations. So are the athletes you want to train, and they're probably a lot more fit than you. Can you make the transition to becoming mentally fit as well? Are you learning and studying your craft so you know everything out there, or are you content to just show your biceps and hope that earns you respect in the gym? Few people cross that bridge successfully, in any endeavor. They think talent is enough. It's not.

MJ understood this better than anyone else. He knew if you were coming to see him play, you were expecting a performance, not just a basketball game. During those championship years, you'd walk up to the old Chicago Stadium or the new United Center, and you knew you were coming to an event. People dressed to be seen, arriving in limos after big, expensive dinners, and those dinners were early because no one wanted to miss a single minute of the show. Every seat was filled during warm-ups, and every time Michael touched the ball, twenty thousand camera flashes went off. It was the toughest ticket in the history of Chicago sports, and every night was like the Oscars. People who had zero interest in sports or the Bulls or basketball paid hundreds of dollars to come to Bulls games, for one reason: to say they had seen Michael Jordan.

How many athletes in any sport, anywhere, can you say that about today?

And while his performance on the court would certainly have been enough to earn him the kind of respect others could only dream of, the real performance started early in the day and didn't end until he was back in the privacy of his home. He made sure the game tickets were organized so he knew where everyone was sitting; he knew what his sponsors needed from him and whom he was supposed to see before and after the game. He paid attention to every single detail, from the tie he chose that day to the way his watchbands matched his shoes. He didn't wear a watch, he wore a "timepiece." He didn't drive a mere car, he drove an "automobile," and he wouldn't get behind the wheel of any vehicle that hadn't just been washed—even when it was raining, the car had to be perfectly clean. Why did he care? Because he knew those crowds around the stadium were packed with people who could never afford a ticket to see him, and this was their one chance, standing outside in the parking lot, to catch a glimpse. For most of his fans, that was as close as they were ever going to get. He was the only player allowed to pull his car directly inside the United Center, but he rarely did; he'd always stop first and get out of the car in plain view of the fans, so all those people could see him. And he maintained that cool composure long after the game, win or lose, until he was back behind closed doors, at home or in his hotel room, where he was free to finally stop and relax. That's when the show ended.

I tell my guys now, just once every few games get out of the car, let the fans take a few pictures, sign a couple of autographs, get back in the car. Takes less than thirty seconds, and those twenty fans who saw you will turn into two hundred, and then two thousand, and pretty soon everyone has a story about seeing you, and now you've touched a lot of lives.

That's how you earn respect. Excellence in everything. Now you're not just another high-paid athlete, you're a class act.

One year I was working with a player going to the Finals, and I was waiting for him in the lobby of the team hotel so we could head to the arena. I'm watching all these players walk out to the bus, and each one looked sloppier than the next. I couldn't believe it. Is this the NBA Finals or are we heading out to rob a liquor store? If Michael had been on that team, he would have pulled every guy off the bus and told them not to come back without a suit and tie. You don't need a $3,000 suit, go to Walmart and buy three for $100, but come back looking like a man, not a kid who got kicked out of school.

And then my guy comes down in the elevator, and he looks worse than anyone else. This is the star of the team, a so-called role model, and he's dressed as if he were going to wash the car. I hustle him into a corner away from the media and lay into him: This is the Finals, this is what you've worked for, you're on the biggest stage where everyone is watching—fans, sponsors, media. This is the ultimate showcase to represent yourself, everything you do here is a reflection on you. What the hell are you thinking?

And he says, No one else is going to put on a suit. I need to fit in with the team. If I wear a suit, I'll stand out.

You probably know this already, but that is not Cleaner talk.

You need to fit in? Really? I thought the whole point was to stand out. You've done all this work to be exceptional, to rise as a superstar, to set the bar higher, and now you want to blend in with everyone else? When you're the guy at the top, you show others how to act, you don't drop down to their level. You command respect and make them measure up to your standards, not the other way around.

You're not here to make friends. You're here because you're the best, and you're not afraid to show it. And if that means setting yourself apart from everyone else, good for you. It means you're doing something right.

Kobe has always set himself apart, quite literally. He shoots alone before the game, never on the same basket as the other guys. And the other players stay away; that's his Zone, and they know it. He might decide to go join them at the other basket, but that's his choice; they would never encroach on his space. That's respect.

When he suffered the shin injury in 2012 and was forced to miss some games, instead of sitting on the bench in sweats or warm-ups as most injured players do, he wore these magnificent suits, carried a clipboard . . . if you didn't know better, you'd think he was the most elegant coach in the history of the NBA, after Chuck Daly. That's how you stand out and set an example. Now you're not just an injured athlete, you're a professional.

I'm not telling you to work at alienating people. But don't be surprised if you do. Coolers are nice; they compensate for their competitive deficiencies by being likable. Cleaners don't have to do that. They set themselves apart from their colleagues and peers, distinguishing themselves by rising to a higher level. When you're completely focused on one thing—your craft—it's hard to pay attention to other people. You might sincerely care about how someone is doing, but you're not going to pick up the phone to find out, and if you do, it's usually because you have a motive for asking. You don't have time for chitchat or lunch or anything that distracts you from your single-minded focus. You don't care about being liked, you care about getting what you want. Not a great way to make and keep friends. But the only way to be truly relentless.

Kobe rarely goes out with teammates, he'd rather work out or watch game film. And he'd much rather have your respect than your friendship. Michael was the same, so was Bird. They relied on their small inner circles of trusted friends—not teammates—who didn't need to be entertained or impressed, people who understood their role in the circle and who shared their friend's vision of success.

You can't get to the top without stepping on some people, but a Cleaner knows where to step without leaving footprints, because you never know when you may need those people again. Being feared doesn't mean being a jerk. I want you to carry yourself so you can be respected, not exposed as an insecure jackass who big-times others so he can feel better about himself. You know that guy: he struts in with an inflated ego and the hot air of cockiness, and leaves behind nothing but the stale air of defeat. That's not a Cleaner, that's a pretender. He might be able to fool a few people for a little while, but when the results are being tallied, he has nowhere to hide.

Cleaners don't make big, bragging announcements about how they topped someone else; they let their results do the talking. Do you think teams are happy when a player calls me in the middle of the season because they've run out of ways to help him? No. Do I care? No. The end result speaks for itself. See the ring on his finger?

I want to be noticed for the excellence of my work, that's all. When people rip me for being an asshole or motherfucker—and they do—to me it means I'm on a level they can't attain or comprehend. That's fear. When others have to fight you by flinging insults, you've already won; it means they have no idea how else to compete with you. Now you know they're intimidated, and you can use it against them every time. The only people not intimidated are others just like you . . . and then it's game on, let's see what you got.

To me, it means nothing when people say they "like" you. Like is average. It leaves no impact, no heat, nothing memorable. It's like being "nice" . . . it's just okay. But it's a million miles from respect, admiration, trust, and an instinctive connection and understanding that you're on the same wavelength and share the same objective.

The greatest compliment to me is "He's an asshole but he's the best at what he does." Thank you. There is no higher praise for a Cleaner. But then you'd better *be* the best at what you do, or you're just an asshole. Can you back it up, or are you just posing?

Cleaner Law: the same guy who is worshipped as a cutthroat competitor is also the guy most likely to be called an asshole by everyone around him. And not just any asshole, but *the* asshole. I'll tell someone he's the biggest asshole I've ever known, and right away he points to another guy and says, "He's a bigger asshole." No, he's not, and you didn't get it: I was giving you a compliment. Take it as a sign that you're doing something right, because if you're truly focused on winning, you're not concerned with friendship or compassion or loyalty, you're not worried about how others will judge you. You know what people say about you, and it just drives you harder. Let them hate you; it only shows their weakness and emotion and makes you more powerful. You don't need friends; your friends need you. You know whom you can trust . . . and they'd better never let you down.

#1. When You're a Cleaner . . .

. . . You trust very few people, and those you trust better never let you down.

Coolers are afraid of the truth because they can't deal with it.
Closers dig for the truth and get upset when it's not in their favor.
Cleaners know when you're lying and wait for the truth to show itself, knowing whatever it is, they'll handle it.

A few years ago I was working with a star who had one of the most legendary entourages in the history of bottle service. A solid entourage is a thing to behold. Basically you have a bunch of unskilled, untrained, generally inexperienced losers from the old neighborhood or some other unknown origin, guys who showed up to a party and never left, all swarming around hoping for a stray piece of ass or a free drink. Then those losers bring around other losers, just to show they know how to party for free. Always free, because none of these bums have a dime in their pockets.

My guys know to never bring the entourage around me because I'll go up to them and say, "Explain to me why you're hanging around here for the next six hours while we're working out. Go read a book, get the car washed, pick up the cleaning, just get out of here, you serve no purpose." And technically, I guess that's false, because they do serve two purposes: telling a superstar how great he is and acting as PHDs—Professional Holders of Dicks. One day I'm going to make PHD T-shirts, congratulate these guys on their accomplishment, and hand them out; those guys will wear anything they get for free.

Until the superstar gets hurt, needs surgery, has to spend a few months rehabbing, and the entire crew slithers off into the night in search of someone new to bank-roll the party.

That's what happened to this guy. One day he's sur-rounded by an entourage of grateful dick holders, the next day he's just got me and an ice bath. No posse, no one kissing his ass, no one to tell him he's the man. For some-one accustomed to calling the shots and having everyone do things his way, it's not easy to give up that kind of con-trol; he's used to telling the team trainers what he will and won't do, and now he's reduced to trusting me to make those decisions for him.

Big-name players can get away with that when they're

dealing with team personnel, because they know they're messing with employees who don't want to jeopardize their jobs and usually have zero leverage to make players do something they don't want to do. I hear it from team trainers all the time: "We tried to do it your way, but he won't do it." No, you couldn't *get* him to do it. If a guy wants to try that with me, we won't be working together for long. You can screw up your own reputation; you're not going to screw up mine.

Our relationship has to be based on trust, or we can't get anywhere. I have a strict protocol for rehabbing specific injuries, and it works. You come to me with complete trust, you follow the rules, or you're wasting your time and mine. And the rules say you don't play until I know you're ready to play, and I'll make that decision based on my experience, not based on your ego or anxiety about getting back in the game.

This player, however, thought he knew better because everyone had always told him he knew better. He did a week of rehab, hobbled onto my basketball court, and declared himself ready to play. "I know my body," he announced. "I'm healthy, I'm playing."

Oh, really? "Listen," I told him, "if you want this to work, you're not getting on a basketball court for another three weeks. You're going to work out with the weights and the underwater treadmill and everything else we can throw at you until we know you're ready, and *then* we'll slowly get you back on the court. But I told you the plan when we started, and we're not going to deviate from the plan."

"Man, you can't keep me from playing," he said.

"You feel that strongly about it?"

"Yeah, that's how strong I feel."

For a moment we just glared at each other. Look, some of these guys are a foot taller than I am, they could toss me across the court. But if you do that, you better make sure I'm dead, because I'm going to get back up and deal with you in ways you cannot begin to comprehend.

"Fine," I said. "Today is your last day here. I can't fix you. I ask three things of anyone who walks in my door: show up, work hard, and listen. If you can't give me all of those three things, I can't help you. You're throwing your money away paying me for a job I can't do." And I left him standing alone with a ball in his hand.

Believe me, I get it. All the media is on your case trying to find out how you're doing, the team is in damage-control mode, the agent is sweating, your family is flipping out, the sponsors want you across the world by the end of the month, you're making payments on five houses and seven cars. Everyone wants to know that the gravy train is still running. That's a lot of pressure.

But I'm still going to make you deal with the truth.

I didn't see him the rest of the day. That night, he called: "Okay. Let's do it." And from that point there wasn't one day that he didn't show up, work hard, and listen.

That's a champion recognizing whom he needed to trust, realizing he didn't have all the answers, and knowing what was at stake if he pretended he did.

In the world of Cleaners, if you can't be trusted, you're

gone. A Cleaner can count on few people, and if you're one of them, it means you've earned it. If you're not, watch your back. A Cleaner never forgives. Or forgets.

But I have to be honest: you should watch your back anyway, because while you can trust a Cleaner to finish the job, if his next job requires him to take you down, you're going down.

I never said a Cleaner was a model citizen. I said he gets results by any means possible. If that makes him a bad guy in your eyes, he can live with that, he doesn't care. You don't have to like him. You just have to trust him to finish what he started.

If you're already a Cleaner, you're probably thinking to yourself, "Trust? Advice? I don't trust anyone and I don't want any advice."

But stay with me here, you need this. And if you're not yet a Cleaner, you need this too. We talked earlier about trusting your instincts to make decisions, and a big part of that is knowing whom you can trust, or whether you can trust anyone at all. Because no matter who you are, part of success means recognizing the people who can help you get where you want to go, putting all the best pieces in place. You have to surround yourself with people who can operate at your level of demanding excellence. You can't be unstoppable, or even great, if you can't do that. And it's probably the hardest thing for a Cleaner to do.

If you're a Cleaner, you already know that when people say, "It's lonely at the top," they're talking about you.

When you've worked so hard and so long to master your craft, learning every detail and nuance of how to do it better than anyone else, inventing and reinventing new ways to set the standard of excellence for yourself and others, who can possibly give you advice on how to still improve? Who's out there to tell you more than you already know? How many people can relate to what you've done, and what you still want to do?

To Cleaners, trusting others is the same as giving up control, and they usually have a painfully hard time with that. Cleaners have this in common: at some point they learned they could only trust themselves. Maybe it was a lesson they learned in childhood, or from something that happened later in life, but it forced them to rely on the sheer power of their gut instinct, and they realized that to survive and succeed, they could never take their hands off the wheel. Once you let someone else drive, they're in control of where you go and how you get there. A Cleaner doesn't sit in the passenger seat unless he's 100 percent confident he can trust the driver, and one thing he knows for sure is that there are a lot of bad drivers out there.

But trust doesn't have to mean giving up control and allowing other people to make decisions for you. Michael was insistent on handling his own responsibilities. He didn't wait for a security guy or a driver or a stylist or a ticket manager to take care of things; he took care of things himself. I'm always amazed to see superstars who can't do anything on their own; they hand over all of their responsibilities to others, and then they're surprised when they don't get the results they wanted.

It's still your responsibility to surround yourself with excellent people and keep those people accountable, which is especially challenging when you're extremely successful. Everyone wants to be part of the action. You have to be careful about whom you choose to keep close, and who needs to find a different day job.

A Cleaner never just hands over responsibility and says, "Here, do this." Too much risk. He'll test you first, maybe for fifteen minutes or fifteen years, whatever it takes, watching how you respond, observing how you work, how you carry yourself, deciding whether your motives and methods are up to his standards. He might not have any need for you now, but when he does, he wants to know whom he can snap into place, and if you've proven yourself, you'll get the call. If not, you're a ghost.

A Cleaner views people as if they're tools, each with unique, indispensable qualities. A hammer can destroy or it can build; a knife in the wrong hands can kill you, but in a doctor's hands it can heal you. A wrench doesn't do the job of a drill, it only does what a wrench is supposed to do. You're only as good as the tools you've chosen, and your ability to use them to their maximum potential.

That's a Cleaner's talent, gathering the best possible assets, placing them exactly where they have to be, and if necessary, moving them into specific situations for his benefit. Cleaners are meticulous about putting their key people in place; they'll take a long time to build that ideal team, but when they finally get everyone they need, they stay committed to keeping the team intact. Think about the most successful people you know. They recognize what works, and they stick with it as long as it keeps working. Cleaners rarely make changes just for the sake of change. What happens when you "shake things up" or "stir the pot"? You get random, unpredictable results. When someone is constantly changing everyone around him, the problem usually isn't those being replaced; more likely, the problem lies with the guy who can't figure out what he needs and wants.

I see a lot of athletes who constantly switch advisers or agents or managers or trainers or assistants; they'll cave in to family pressure to hire the brother-in-law to do a job he can't handle, or they decide to save some money and use an old pal to manage the books. Pretty soon no one's working together, everyone is bitter and annoyed, and instead of taking pressure off the player so he can focus on the job that keeps everything else afloat, now he's got to manage personnel problems. I look around at the inevitable mess that follows and I think, "This is your business. What are you doing?" The whole team has to have one goal so we can all reach that end result together: it can't be about individual priorities. A good team looks at everything: Should we be making this appearance or attending that function, or do we need to be working out or practicing or getting healthy? The Cleaner has to be able to trust that everyone around him has his back and isn't operating under some separate agenda. When you're an A+ person, you want A+ people around you, and everyone has to be accountable for doing A+ work.

And part of making the Cleaner look good is having

the balls to tell him the truth, even when he doesn't want to hear it.

When someone says, "I need to be surrounded by positive people," I just laugh. You know what that really means? *I want people who will lie to my face and make me feel better.* You didn't hire me to tell happy, shiny lies, my job is to set people straight, no matter what the consequence. And if that makes me sound cold or harsh, I'm fine with that. It's made me very good at what I do.

A player has so many people giving him advice; what can I say to him that he'll really hear, what's the one thing he never thought of, the thing that makes a difference? How can I make it more powerful than the hundred things he's heard before?

Again: the truth is simple.

During halftime, I sometimes meet Kobe in the tunnel before he goes out for the second half. I talk, he listens. It takes less than fifteen seconds. What I say to him is between us, but you can be sure he knows it's the truth.

All I've ever done with these guys is give them a few phrases or an idea that makes them stop in their tracks. That's it. Then let them figure it out. That way it's their idea.

That's my relationship with Dwyane as well. After his simultaneous knee and shoulder surgeries in 2007, I sent him back to Miami ready to play and remained in regular contact with the Heat's training staff to make sure he was staying on track. One day I get a call from them: Can I come down to Miami and talk to Dwyane? Sure. I get there and the staff tells me they want him to do A, B, C, and D.

Got it. Let me talk to him. I sit down with Dwyane: I need you to do A, B, and C. Forget D. Okay? Okay. I'm there for eight minutes. Get back on the plane and go home. The next day they call me: "Hey, he did A, B, and C!" Of course he did. That's trust. I don't need to be the center of things, I just want to do my job and get out of the way. If I'm doing it right, I'm always around and you'll never see me.

The truth is simple. It requires no explanation, analysis, rationale, or excuse; it's just a simple statement that leaves no doubt. You can look at it from every angle, hold it up to the light, flip it over, slice it up, smash it with an ax . . . it's still the truth. But highly successful people rarely get to hear the truth; they're surrounded by assistants and security and aides and the PHDs who go to tremendous lengths to keep their place in the circle of trust by managing the truth, shoveling polite opinions and puffy compliments, and generally keeping the boss happy.

But the boss doesn't always need to be happy. Sometimes he needs an honest smack in the head. You want to be the most valuable guy in the circle? Be the one who looks the Cleaner straight in the eye and tells him what everyone else is afraid to say. He might hate it, and hate you for saying it, but a true Cleaner knows when he's being bullshitted and when he's being set straight. And guaranteed, the next time he needs to know whom he can trust, he'll be looking for you.

But if you expect the truth from me, you'd better give me the truth in return. Before I ask a question, I already know the answer. And I'll keep asking until you give me the truth.

You been drinking a lot?

No.

Not drinking?

No.

Because your body looks like you've been drinking.

No.

How often are you drinking?

I'm not dri—

Don't even answer, I already know. You need a thirty-day program. If you don't do it, your career is over. You don't want to do it? Up to you. But you need it.

You can't make things better until you stop making things worse. In business, in sports, doesn't matter, this isn't personal. Every year I get coaches and agents and GMs calling me for an opinion, and I appreciate that they value my input. *Can he play?* No. *But did you see what he did at . . .* No. *But if we can get him healthy . . .* No. Let me save you a whole lot of money and grief and anxiety, he can't play.

When the answer is no, a Cleaner says no; he doesn't soften it or wrap it in something pretty. No excuses, and no explanation afterward. Explanations are another way of saying, "I wasn't sure, but then I went through this whole, long thought process until I came to a decision, and now I'm pretty sure. I hope you understand." And if you do need to explain, do so knowing you're opening the door to further discussion, because when the other guy sees you had some indecision, he's going to try to negotiate. *No* is a closed door, no negotiation. Someone asks you to do something you don't want to do, and you start explaining, that person is going to ask you again and again and again. Don't explain, don't make excuses. Truth takes one sentence. Simple and direct. A question, an answer.

Attaining excellence means finding those answers, not just settling for the convenient, easy route. It means seeking and accepting the truth, and adapting as necessary. How many times do you see a player rush back from an injury, only to be injured worse? More often than not, the trainer knew what he was doing, and the player either panicked or didn't trust him or listened to bad advice from people who had no idea what they were talking about. Your back feels better? That's great. How about everything connected to your back, you want to take care of that too? Or should we wait until you reinjure it in two weeks?

Athletes are surrounded by an endless parade of experts on everything; they have coaches, trainers, doctors, agents, advisers, wives, parents, and, yes, the dick holders. Everyone has an opinion. By the time a player gets to me, he's lost touch with his precious instincts, and when I tell him what we're going to do to fix his game or mend his body, he's usually hearing things no one else has told him. I have my methods, and I know they work. Let me do this, I tell him. Tough call for a star athlete used to getting his way and doing what he wants.

Whether you're an athlete, an entrepreneur, a CEO, a rock star, or you're just starting out in life, know what you know, and what you don't know. Most of the time when we ask for advice, we don't want the truth. We want the answer we're seeking. Be open to advice that goes against what you want.

Cleaner Law: surround yourself with those who want you to succeed, who recognize what it takes to be successful. People who don't pursue their own dreams probably won't encourage you to pursue yours; they'll tell you every negative thing they tell themselves.

Cleaners trust few people; they'd almost always rather follow their instincts and fix the situation later if they're wrong, than trust someone else and kick themselves for not listening to that voice inside. If a Cleaner screws up, he wants it to be because he did what he thought was right, not because he did what someone else told him to do.

On the other hand, when a Cleaner trusts you, he'll stay out of your way and let you do your job without critique or interference, especially if you're a Cleaner as well, because the only thing he cares about are those final results. He doesn't care how you do it, just do it.

But he has to trust you first.

Michael and Phil were both extreme Cleaners. Michael trusted Phil to let him do his thing, and Phil trusted Michael to do it. Phil would tell him, Look, just start running the triangle, then do whatever you have to do, but at least run it so it looks like we're running *something*. And Michael would run a few plays, then take care of business his own way. End result? It worked.

But when it doesn't work, and two Cleaners go their separate ways, they both know for sure it's never over. The competitive drive is so strong that they never stop battling for supremacy. Beware of the Cleaner you cut loose; he'll be back, and he'll be stronger than he ever was.

When a Cooler speaks, you have doubts.
When a Closer speaks, you listen.
When a Cleaner speaks, you believe.

A Cleaner can listen to others and still make his own decisions . . . collecting information, processing it, deciding. When Michael and I started together, we were both learning and figuring it out. He knew basketball, I knew the human body. I didn't question his authority and he didn't question mine. But now I'm the teacher; these guys call me for advice on everything: their kids, their baby-mama drama, how should they handle everything you can think of. They trust me. Why? Because I give them a straight answer. Few words have as much impact as *trust me*. If you say that to someone, you're taking on some serious responsibility, and you'd better be able to deliver. So when they come to me and say, "Yeah, I did this," they know I'm going to help. I might first shake my head and say, "You honestly thought you'd get away with that?" But we're going to find a way to deal with it and minimize the damage.

If I say something they don't like—which is pretty often—it's for their benefit. Always for them. If there's a choice between being the asshole who tells them things are about to go bad, or the good buddy who lies to their faces and tells them everything is great, guess what: I'll be the asshole who keeps them from failing. They're used to people showering them with roses, and I'm bringing the thorns.

#1. When You're
a Cleaner . . .

. . . You don't recognize failure; you know there's more than one way to get what you want.

A Cooler accepts what he can't do and gives up.
A Closer recognizes what he can't do but keeps working at it.
A Cleaner knows what he can do and stays with it until he decides to do something else.

On the night the Chicago Bulls were eliminated from the 1995 NBA playoffs by the Orlando Magic, I sat with Michael in the darkened United Center until 3:00 a.m. He had just returned to basketball two months earlier, following his first retirement and brief baseball career; so much had happened in the last year.

Dressed in his suit and tie, he looked around the brand-new arena that had replaced the legendary Chicago Stadium earlier that season and said, "I hate this fucking building."

"You built this fucking building," I said.

During that series, some of the Orlando players said he didn't look like the old #23, which he didn't; he was wearing #45, he wasn't ready, and I knew it better than anyone else. His endurance, his shot . . . there just hadn't been enough time to get him back to the level of excellence that people had grown accustomed to.

Predictably, there was plenty of talk about how his baseball career had failed, his basketball comeback had failed, he had failed. Michael Jordan was done, they said.

And as usual, they were wrong. A Cleaner is done when *he* says he's done, not when you say he's done.

In fact, you saying it usually ensures the opposite.

At the end of that game, he had a message for the Magic as the all players shook hands and left the court: *Enjoy this win, 'cause it ain't gonna happen again.*

Then he changed his number back to #23, and the following season he led the Bulls to an NBA-record 72 wins and the first of three more championship rings to go with the three he'd already won before he "failed."

Failed? How can you fail when your worst day is better than most people's best?

I don't understand the concept of failure.

If you don't succeed at everything you do on your first attempt, does that mean you "failed"? Isn't it a good thing that you keep coming back and working at it until you succeed? How can that be failure?

What most people think of as failure, a Cleaner sees as an opportunity to manage and control a situation, pulling it around to his advantage, doing something everyone else says is impossible. If there's a 2 percent chance that something will work, and a 98 percent chance that it won't, he'll take the 98 percent risk just to show he took the challenge and did what everyone else said couldn't be done. It may take years, and all kinds of work no one else will ever see, but eventually a Cleaner is going to own that situation and make it work to his advantage. He has to; it's the only way he knows. This didn't work, so let's do that. If that doesn't work, we can do this. How many ways can you prepare? How many different pathways can you create so you don't eventually run into a ditch? And even if you do run into the ditch, how many options do you have for getting out?

It fascinates me to hear the criticism of Michael as the owner and GM of the Charlotte Bobcats. After four years as a minority partner, Michael took control in 2010 and became the first former player to become the majority owner of an NBA team. Cleaner Law: if your name is on the door, you'd better control what goes on behind that door.

Right away, the critics pounced on the team's poor performance, questioning whether the Bobcats' failure would tarnish Michael's legacy, and comparing him to other players who had made the leap to management. "Larry Bird! Joe Dumars! Jerry West!" Great executives who did great things with the teams they worked for, but that's the difference: they all worked for someone else. Michael is working for himself. It's his money, his name on that door. There's a big difference between being hired for a job that you'll eventually leave, voluntarily or involuntarily, and owning the business, which has never before been done in the NBA by a former player. How can you fail at something that's never been done, when there's no previous measure of success?

After a terrible 2011–12 season, he blamed no one, took full responsibility for the team's situation, and said he was going to figure it out. Probably doesn't help that the team's best player is actually its owner. But when Michael says, "I never want to be in the record books for failure," as he told reporters after the season, believe him.

Let's make this simple: Failure is what happens when you decide you failed. Until then, you're still always looking for ways to get to where you want to be.

It's Derek Jeter responding to a reporter who asked if the Yankees were panicking during a late-season slump, and how Jeter was dealing with it: "I don't panic so I don't have to deal with it." Total Cleaner. Or Dallas Cowboys tight end Jason Witten, offering to sign a medical waiver so he could return to action with a lacerated spleen, against doctors' orders. It's Dwyane refusing to go down with that bad knee in the playoffs, or Kobe refusing to sit out with multiple injuries—including the concussion— that would have staggered anyone else. That's how you decide to not fail. You go, and you go, always looking for the unexpected option that keeps the situation in your control.

Success and failure are 100 percent mental. One person's idea of success might seem like a complete failure to someone else. You must establish your own vision of what it means to be unstoppable; you can't let anyone else define that for you. What does your gut tell you? What do your instincts know about what you should be doing, how you're going to succeed, and what you're going to succeed at? How can anyone tell you what that should be?

When someone else says you've failed, what they really mean is "If that were me, I would feel like a failure." Well, that guy's not you, and he's obviously not a Cleaner, because Cleaners don't recognize failure.

I understand the challenge of fighting back against all odds while others want you to fail. When I built the Attack Athletics facility in Chicago in 2007, I had already been in business for almost twenty years. I had already worked with the best athletes in the world, traveled to places and seen things others can only dream of, and I wanted to take Attack Athletics to the next level. Everyone said it was the final stage in my evolution as a trainer. But to me, it was just the beginning. I built a state-of-the-art athletic-training facility that brought people from all over the world, a place that no other individual trainer could ever have dreamed of building and owning.

I had certain expectations and plans, and they all came to fruition; the new venture was everything I wanted it to be. But as with any business, unexpected situations force you to make adjustments, and I was faced with difficult decisions that would change the direction of the facility. Players facing the NBA lockout didn't want to make the financial investment in their training without the certainty of a season. My major clients—Kobe, Dwyane, and many others—understandably wanted me wherever they were, so I was all over the world with them while my building was sitting in Chicago. Hard way to run a business. And before long, there was some buzz about the "failure" of Attack Athletics.

What happened with the building was a setback. But dealing with setbacks is how you achieve success. You learn, and you adapt. When everyone else is talking about how you "failed," you show up like a professional, remap your course, and get back to work. That's the progression of good-great-unstoppable. No one starts at unstoppable. You fuck up, you figure it out, you trust yourself.

Let me say this: Attack Athletics is who I am and what I do, it's not a building. The building was about equipment and environment and a revolutionary concept. Attack Athletics is me, and my training philosophy, and it goes wherever I go. Attack Athletics is the work I do all over the world, and I work hard to be sure that my clients and I don't fail at anything we do. We always find a way to make it work.

But when you're the best at anything, you wear a big target on your back. When your colleagues and friends and enemies start talking and sniping behind your back, you know you've done something right if they care that much about you and your business, and whether you're going to "lose." Lose? What I lose you never had.

A Cleaner never sees failure because to him it's never over. If something doesn't go as planned, he instinctively looks for options to make things work a different way. He doesn't feel embarrassed or ashamed, he doesn't blame anyone else, and he doesn't care what anyone else says about his situation. It's never the end, it's never over.

And he knows, without a doubt, that whatever happens, he'll find a way to come out on top. If you ever find me and a bear wrestling in the woods, help the bear.

Make the choice to turn "failure" into success. If your team doesn't win a championship, if your business falls apart, if you don't achieve something you worked for, move to the next step in your evolution. Remember who you are, and how you got this far. Listen to your gut. What is it telling you?

It's never over. You have choices:

The Cooler admits defeat.

The Closer works harder.

The Cleaner strategizes for a different outcome.

Admitting defeat has no place in this discussion, or in this book, because the words *quit* and *relentless* just don't work together in any productive way. People who admit defeat and say they had no choice just aren't serious about success, excellence, or themselves. They say they'll "try" and then give up when that doesn't work.

Fuck "try." Trying is an open invitation to failure, just another way of saying, "If I fail, it's not my fault, I tried."

You *tried* your best? Or did you *do* your best? Huge difference. "Well, I tried." Okay, now tell me what you *did*.

Do, or don't do.

Do it, and if it doesn't work, do it again.

Did you do it this way? That way? Did you explore every idea you had? Is there anything else you could possibly do to turn things in your favor?

If you aim at excellence, you have to be willing to sacrifice. That is the price of success. You never know how bad you want it until you get that first bitter taste of not getting it, but once you taste it, you're going to fight like hell to get that bitterness out of your mouth. Maybe you got benched, or you lost a lot of money, or someone else got the promotion you wanted. Others might give up, and they'll be the first to say you should give up too. But did you stop because you wanted to, or because they told you to? Is there still work to be done? Do you still feel the anger inside you, driving you to take action and turn things around? A Closer will keep going until he's forced to stop—remember, he's called a Closer because he's there at the end. But once the end arrives, he knows it, he feels it. It's over.

A Cleaner can't ever accept that it's over. But he does recognize when it's time to change direction.

One of the hardest things to do is to change course once you've set your goals. You made a decision, you worked for it, you earned the payoff . . . but for whatever reason, it's not going the way you planned.

It's not weak to recognize when it's time to shift directions.

It's weak to refuse to consider other options and fail at everything because you couldn't adapt to anything.

We've all been there: you just know something's not

right. Maybe you're not advancing as quickly as you planned, or you're not making the money you anticipated, or maybe you just don't like what you're doing or whom you're doing it with. Or maybe events outside of your control have impacted your situation.

This is where instinct is the most valuable tool you can possibly possess, because only you can decide whether to hear what the voice inside is telling you.

In pro sports, it's the decision to retire or to take a shot at one more season. For a young athlete, it's deciding whether to sit on the bench or to find a new sport to play. In business, it can be the choice to change careers or jobs, start or sell a business. In any situation, it's the courage and confidence to know it's time to make a change.

It takes a special person to say enough is enough and know when it's time to start redirecting your effort into something that can succeed. Maybe your dream isn't going to play out the way you originally envisioned it, but with some creativity and vision you can redirect your goals toward something that keeps you connected to what you always wanted.

I can tell myself with no hesitation that I'm the best at what I do. I earned it. But to become the best, I had to learn a lot of lessons about always being prepared to change direction, and refusing to get sucked into other people's opinions of what it means to succeed or fail.

The first time I learned that lesson, I was a basketball player at University of Illinois–Chicago with big dreams and a torn ACL. A botched rehab led to hip issues, leg issues, more knee issues. I have more orthopedic issues than you can imagine. I had no idea at that time that my greatest weakness would become my greatest strength, that experiencing every possible injury and surgery would allow me to help others to deal with the same, at the most elite level.

I was a pretty good player, but not NBA caliber. I just wasn't ready to admit it. When I suffered that first injury, all I wanted to do was play basketball. I'm not the most religious person, but to me, the torn ACL was a message saying, "Listen, you're spending too much time trying to work on this game, it's not going to happen. So let's just bust up your knee so you can focus on what you're supposed to do with your life and get you on the right path faster."

But I wasn't ready to look at a different ending for my dream. I kept playing, wearing a big brace on my messed-up knee, and trying to overcome the aftermath of the injury and disastrous rehab.

Then one day, the turning point: I was playing in a tournament, and this kid I didn't even know came up to me and said: "I remember when you were good."

Oh.

Got it.

That was the wake-up call, the message I needed to realize I was forcing a situation that had no chance of succeeding. It wasn't about the kid's comment; he was only saying what I already knew. I just hadn't accepted it yet. I played in one pickup game after that, and that was it.

It was time to find a new ending for that dream.

Learn. Adapt. I realized if my damaged body couldn't

help me play basketball, I would use what I'd learned and find a way to turn it into something positive. And I could already see what it was: I didn't want to work for a team, I wanted to work for myself, take someone in basketball and make him better than he was before. That was how I would make my mark on the NBA.

I guess it worked.

Of course, it took me a little longer to figure how that dream was actually going to take shape. I was still chasing Brad Sellers and the rest of the Bulls, writing them all letters, offering my training services. No one responded. I assumed Michael Jordan would be the least likely to hire a trainer, especially one who had never trained a professional athlete, so I never even contacted him.

That's how I learned: Don't try. *Do*.

Today I teach the best of the best to take care of their bodies because when I hit initial roadblocks, I refused to see my situation as a failure. You take what everyone else sees as a negative and turn it to your advantage. You don't sulk, you don't curl up and die, you glare at it and think, if it's not going to happen this way, it's sure as hell going to happen that way. And you tell anyone who doubts you, "I got this."

Just don't expect everyone else to understand or agree with your new plan. Most people are either content to stay with the safe thing, or they're too scared to leave a bad thing, and they'll put all that fear and doubt on you. They anticipate failure; you anticipate opportunity. When I decided to go into this field, everyone said, "Oh, a gym teacher." No. "Personal trainer?" No. I am not a personal trainer. A personal trainer meets you at the gym for an hour, helps you with your workout, and sees you the next time you want an appointment. I work for my clients seven days a week, 365 days a year, around the clock. You need me, I'm there. You can call me an architect, or an athletic specialist. An architect constructs a building, I construct a body, from the inside out. How do I rebuild that shoulder? How do I structure that physique so it's stronger and more durable and powerful than ever before? I'm a physical architect, responsible for every fiber of that mind and body you've entrusted to me.

All because I "failed" as a basketball player.

To me, success isn't about how much money I can make; it's never been about that. Success is about doing things that no one else can do.

A couple of years ago, I spent the summer working with Robbie Hummel, who was playing for Purdue, a great kid who had just torn his ACL for the second time in eight months. The first time, in 2010, he was a junior with just eight games left in the season and was already considered one of the top players in the country. Determined to get back to the game, he went through surgery and rehab with trainers at school and returned to the Boilermakers the following season for his senior year, ready to play.

At the very first team practice, he tore the ACL again. Out for the season, and possibly forever.

Two surgeries in eight months? Returning from a double ACL injury? That's a lot of work for an uncertain outcome. There was talk that the promising career of the 6'8" All-American forward might be over. That's when his dad called me; could I get him back to where he needed to be, so he could have one more shot as a fifth-year senior?

I don't know anyone else in my business who has successfully rehabbed even one double ACL injury, but Robbie would be my third. I knew what we'd have to do for him; it would take months of commitment and serious mental toughness. His choice.

For seven months, he worked on that rehab, five days a week, twice a day, at the Attack Athletics facility in Chicago and also back at school in Valparaiso. He'd drive an hour each way to see us, and I think he was a little stunned by how fast and hard we put him to work. "The first day I figured they'd talk to me and take my height and weight," he told reporters. "Within an hour they had me puking in a trash can."

Our goal was to have him at full strength by the start of Big Ten conference play for the 2011–12 season. People said it was impossible. His surgeon had cleared him to play, but he still had one test to pass for me before I'd give him the green light—the forty-eight-inch jump down to the floor and back up. Same test I give all my guys after knee/ankle/hip rehab. The day he finally achieved that was the day we said good-bye and sent him back to school, good to go. Our job was done and his was just beginning.

Not only did he return to the game better than ever, he went on to be named First Team All–Big Ten for the third time in his career, ranking in the top ten for scoring, rebounds, blocks, 3-pointers, and free throws. And in his final appearance in the NCAA tournament, he dominated with 26 points, including five 3-pointers, in a narrow loss to Kansas. By then we were no longer working together, but I was so pleased for him when he was drafted in the second round of the NBA draft and then headed to Spain to start his professional career.

Where he promptly tore his meniscus.

More surgery, more work, more commitment.

A lot of guys would quit. He kept going.

It's all a choice. I tell my athletes everything up front and let them decide whether to keep fighting or give up. Tracy McGrady was facing an eighteen-month process to rehab his knee, and he had to make a tough choice: Are you willing to give up two years of your career so when you're forty or fifty you'll still have a perfect knee . . . or are you willing to take a chance and cut those eighteen months in half, work for a superstrong knee that's going to last you through your whole career, and deal with the remaining issues when you're done playing? That's not a decision I can make for him. But no one ever chooses the longer rehab.

In these cases, I offer choices, and the athletes have to decide what they want to do. You can be good by playing it safe. You can't be relentless unless you're willing to take chances. Safe makes you good, chances make you great.

Gilbert Arenas is another who decided to take the chance with his body. I told him, you have about a hundred degrees flexion in this knee. Three years from now you're going to have about ninety degrees. Seven years from now, maybe seventy-five. Gil's question: How much flexion do I need to play? I said around forty-five. He said, Okay, I'm good. We knew we could get Gilbert back 100 percent because any individual who's willing to pack up all his stuff and relocate to Chicago to spend three months being tortured by me is already in the right frame of mind.

Those huge decisions ultimately determine success or failure. Whom do they trust? The doctors have to give the full medical opinion for a complete recovery. They're going to treat your symptoms; I'm going to overcome the cause. The teams and sponsors want the guys back on the floor as fast as possible. The agents are thinking about how to play the situation so it works for the next contract. I just look at the damage, talk to everyone, and give the guy his options. If you do this, you get this; if you do that, you get that. Here's what caused the injury, here's what we'll do so it doesn't happen again. Your call.

Being trusted with those life-altering, high-stakes decisions is what makes me feel successful. Money is nice, but it's better to help someone who doesn't have much time left to excel at something. I love a guy like Juwan Howard, who came into the league in 1994 and for almost twenty years worked his ass off year-round for the opportunity to get a ring, which he finally achieved with the Heat in 2012. You know how much work that takes in your late thirties, to stay in condition and keep making those teams, just because you refuse to go down without that ultimate prize? That's a guy who refused to accept failure and came away a winner.

With athletes, you have to realize that every day brings them closer to the end of their careers, closer to that decision about whether to walk away or go harder. How can I enhance whatever time they have left so they can be successful? That's where I look for my success.

They all want it to last forever and see the end of their careers as some kind of loss. But it doesn't have to be, if they've put the pieces in place ahead of time. I've had this conversation over and over with guys nearing the end of their careers: In one year you're going to be irrelevant. You'll leave a legacy as a player, but what does that mean when you get up every day with nothing to do? Figure it out now, before you're just another ex-player looking for attention. Your shoe deal won't last forever, and only so many guys are going to be able to coach or sit in the broadcast booth. What's your plan? How do you turn this great career into something even greater, so you can continue to be unstoppable for years to come? Do it now, because if you wait too long, those other options start slipping away. Other people are chasing the same ideas, and they're getting ahead of you while you cling to this old thing that's not working.

A Cleaner knows when to walk away, and which direction to walk. Never running, always walking; he leaves smoothly and on his own terms. He can lose a battle because he's still planning to win the war. Lose a game, but win the season. Lose a season, come back and win the next three. Lose a job, start a new business. No one else is getting the last word on whether he succeeded.

#1. WHEN YOU'RE
A CLEANER . . .

. . . You don't celebrate your achievements because you always want more.

A Cooler is first to arrive at the celebration and last to leave.
A Closer will make an appearance, then go out with his own crew.
A Cleaner just wants to get back to work.

I'm not here for the parade. By the time my client wakes up the next day drenched in party sweat and a champagne-soaked victory T-shirt, I'm long gone.

We'll find each other for a couple minutes when it's all over, and that's it.

"You good?"

"I'm good."

Done.

Next.

A Cleaner's favorite words.

There's always more work to do. And more to prove. Always more to prove.

Let everyone else celebrate. You're still not satisfied.

If you won in six, you're disappointed you didn't win in five. If you benched 195, why not 200? If you made a deal for a million dollars, you'll keep wondering if you could have done it for $1.2 million.

Never satisfied.

On the rare occasions when you do feel like celebrating, it's a brief, private moment you don't share with anyone else, because no one could possibly understand what you went through to get to that point. The others can celebrate because you made it all possible. They may not even realize that, but you do.

Everything you accomplished, everything you worked for, you didn't do any of it for the celebration, and you didn't do it for anyone else. You did it for that exquisite moment, that electrifying, powerful surge of satisfaction that everyone dreams about but few ever get to experience.

Yet the minute you experience it, it's already fading. And all you can think about is doing whatever it takes to get it back.

It's that momentary feeling of *"Enough,"* followed by a deep, hot surge of *"More."*

A Cleaner knows the quiet melancholy of victory. While everyone else enjoys the win, he waits for the impending letdown, the unyielding reminder that the glory is already in the past, and there's a new challenge ahead, bigger and harder and more grueling than whatever he just completed.

If you want to find the Cleaner at a victory party, look for the guy standing off to the side by himself, watching everyone else. He's happy for them because they can go home feeling that their work is complete. But his is always just beginning. He's already thinking about the next move, the next risk, the next kill. Watch Pat Riley the next time he wins a title; no one looks more subdued at a celebration. He knows too well what it took to get there and what has to be done to stay there.

A true Cleaner is at his lowest soon after he reaches his highest. For five minutes, he's completely exhilarated. For the next twenty-four hours, he's relatively happy. After that . . . what?

Back to work.

Everyone else will tell him he did a great job, and he knows it's true. But their approval means nothing to him because the standards he sets for himself are so much higher than anyone else can possibly set for him. Win or lose, all he thinks about is how he could have done it better or smoother or faster or some way other than how he did it. So the job gets done, but he's still always thinking about how he could have done more.

That's the relentless pursuit of excellence, always believing in your ability, demanding more of yourself than anyone else could ever ask of you.

Winning is an addiction. The great Vince Lombardi

once said, "Winning is a habit," which is also true, but I think it's a habit that inevitably becomes the addiction. You can't understand it until you taste it, and then you can spend a lifetime craving more. You feel it in your gut, in the dull ache of your dark side begging for it. When you're alone in the Zone, you know nothing except the unwavering hunger for success. Every choice you make, every sacrifice, every moment you spent alone preparing and learning and dreaming . . . it's all to feed that addiction.

And if you ever once feel the need to question why it's necessary to work so hard or wonder if it's all worth it . . . just go ahead and quit. You don't get it.

It's hard to describe the enormity of winning when it's combined with the realization that to repeat the experience you have to start all over again, go through the whole process, and work even harder for an uncertain outcome. When I first started working with Kobe, Juwan Howard went up to him after a game to say he'd been working with me for a long time and talked about how I had helped his longevity. Then he asked Kobe how many more years he wanted to play.

"Until I get number six," Kobe said.

He didn't answer in years, which was what Juwan asked, and he didn't answer by age or the length of his contract, which is how most players address that question. He answered in rings. He already had three at that point. He got two more the following seasons. As I write this, he needs one more to reach his goal. Two more if I have anything to say about it.

That's the addiction. Others think about how many

years are left on their contracts, or how many seasons are left in their worn-down bodies. The great ones don't even consciously think about it. There's just one automatic response: win. They don't think about if or when they'll hit their ceiling, they don't believe they have a ceiling. They just keep going, and they leave on their own terms, when they want to, not when anyone else tells them to.

A few years ago I was working with a player trying to come back after surgery, and he said to me, "I just want to get better so I can get even with everybody."

That got my attention. "Say that again," I said.

"I just want to get even with everyone."

"Define *even*," I said.

"I want to get back at all these people who said I couldn't do it."

"You know what *even* means?" I asked. "It means you're equal to them, right next to them. Side by side." Silence. "Do you truly want to get even with everyone, or do you really want to get ahead of them? Why stand next to anyone when you can push beyond them? In the game of basketball, you get around someone so you can get past them. Play this game the same way. You go for the win, you don't settle for a tie."

He got it. Not everyone does. Think about the people you know who are so talented and gifted and capable, yet completely void of the ability to advance, as if an invisible cap were over them. Most people allow themselves to be limited that way, either by what others tell them or what they think of themselves, and they decide they can settle for whatever they have under that cap. My job is to get you to bump up that cap. In everything you do, I want you better and stronger than the last time you did it. When a player comes to me and says, "I'm gonna get a triple double tonight," and then he goes out and gets the triple double and everyone gets all excited, all I can think is, "What was stopping you last night?"

A Cleaner performs for himself, and everyone else wins. Whatever he does to satisfy his goals internally transfers to them externally. When he achieves what he desires, everyone else around him benefits. If he's the boss and his company makes a massive profit because he worked around the clock maneuvering a huge deal, his employees win. He's the guy who hits the game-winning shot because he practiced that damn shot a thousand times every single fucking day, and his teammates get to go home winners. But they'll celebrate and he won't because he'll be looking at the stat sheet, skimming over the positive stuff and going straight to the negative. "Thirty points, ten assists . . . damn, two turnovers." And that's all he's going to remember: "Oh, the night I had two turnovers." He played a near-perfect game, but to him, not perfect enough.

The drive to close the gap between near-perfect and perfect is the difference between great and unstoppable. You never shake the uneasy feeling that you can't ever be satisfied with your results; you always believe you could have done better, and you stop at nothing to prove it. Is it an ideal way to live? I don't know. It's not easy, that's for sure. You hope your family and friends ultimately understand. They might not. Your whole life is essentially dedicated to one goal, to the exclusion of everything else. Whether you're focused on business, sports, relationships, anything, you have to be committed to saying, "I'm doing this, I'll give up whatever I have to give up so I can do this, I don't care what anyone thinks, and if there are consequences that affect the other parts of my life, I'll deal with them when I have to."

That's Kobe: everything he does is all about excellence. Everything. Nothing else matters. You hear people say that all the time, "I'll do whatever it takes!"—but he truly lives it. Every detail of his life, every hour of his day, the lonely time he spends in the gym, the people he seeks out to help him maintain that excellence, everything revolves around being on top and staying there. That's why we work so well together; he has one focus and I have one focus: our shared addiction to winning. And everything we do is about that one objective.

But when you're never satisfied, life can be lonely. People think success will make them happy, but when you experience it, it's usually different from what you imagined. You'll have what you desire, but be prepared for the possibility that you'll be standing alone because you had the balls to take the unpopular path and you went to extremes that others won't ever understand. You'll finally have everything you ever dreamed of, but now you'll know for sure what you suspected all along: Nobody else understands what you went through, or what you did to get there.

To me, never being satisfied means being prepared for any situation, ready to adapt seamlessly without panic or fluster. It means scrutinizing every detail, paying meticulous attention to things no one else would even notice. I don't have to watch the ball go into the basket, I know from looking at the shot whether it's going in. That's my job, to show you why your wrist needs to be here and your elbow needs to be there, why this shot isn't working and that shot is perfect. I show my players how it all works together, and they can't believe it. That's what separates me from anyone else: I never overlook the details, and I'll make sure you don't either.

But when you live and work that way, it can take its toll, and one of the biggest challenges facing highly competitive people is burnout. You win that prize, you make your money, you get the glory . . . it can be awfully tempting to lie down and let someone else carry the load for a while. The pressure, the scrutiny, the strain on your personal life—it affects just about everyone. If you work in anything other than sports, you have options. Change jobs, change careers, take a sabbatical, go back to school, learn a new part of your business. In sports? Forget it, unless your talent and skills are so extreme that you can afford the time away, such as Michael going to play baseball. To me, that's what made him the greatest: he had the ability to control time when he was in the Zone, and he was always in the Zone. He left and returned, refined his basketball skills, and it was as if nothing had changed. But otherwise, athletes don't have the luxury of time; they only get a few short years to leave their mark, and they're done before most people their age are just getting started.

At some point, though, every elite athlete just gets

tired of putting in the relentless work it takes to be exceptional. It's especially common with athletes who become successful at a young age, such as tennis players and Olympians, who feel they never got the chance to be kids because they were always working and training and traveling and competing. If you never had a chance to be a kid, you want that for yourself, because it's completely instinctive to want to have fun, ignore the rules, and just forget about responsibility and goals and performance. I get that. But I'm convinced childhood is overrated; you can have a much better childhood as an adult, when you have the freedom and the affluence to enjoy it. You get this small window to be a legend, and you have the rest of your life to act like a kid, at any age. Push it as far as you can, and even if you make it until you're thirty or thirty-five, you still have decades ahead to enjoy what you built for yourself.

Some athletes know they're done, and that's it. But when that burnout hits a guy who isn't done, it's extremely hard for him to find his way back to where he was. Maybe he won a title, took it easy during the off-season, and returned the next year feeling a little content and satisfied. Usually, only one thing can bring him back: the competitive spirit, the idea that someone else is about to take what's his, the realization that while he was content to get fat and lazy, everyone else was still lean and hungry. Then he has to get busy playing catch-up, or he won't be the champ for long.

In Michael's Hall of Fame induction speech, I heard him say something that made me think, "I thought we were done, but now I'm not really sure." I'm still not sure. I'll be ready just in case.

A Cleaner feels burnout like everyone else, but the idea of walking away and not thinking about what he walked away from creates more anxiety and stress than keeping it going; that addiction is still demanding to be fed. That's why you see guys retire and return; they're still not satisfied, and they still have something to prove. Not to you, but to themselves. The pressure is all internal.

You have to crave that pressure, embrace it, and never let up.

You don't have to love it. You just have to be insatiable for the results.

• • •

I've accomplished and experienced enough "impossible" things to realize that nothing is impossible, and every day I crave the challenge of proving that. It's why I only train athletes and not Hollywood celebrities: everything I do is about performance, and when my guys step out there, there's no makeup, no script, no hiding. Whatever happens, it's out there for everyone to see. Actors and actresses can have their flaws and mistakes airbrushed and edited out; my guys have nowhere to hide. I love that pressure. I love getting these athletes ready to go, and seeing all our hard work turn into a masterpiece with the world watching. I loved getting Michael in shape to play baseball, and then back into basketball shape so he could win three more rings to go with the first three. Loved taking Kobe to the highest level and beyond, so he could chase his dream for that fourth and fifth championship and still keep going for more. Loved running into Pat Riley the night Miami won the 2012 championship and having him ask me how I got Dwyane so explosive in just a few short days. You give me a situation, I will make it work. That's what drives me. A new challenge every time, a new way to do things better than we did before.

I'll admit, it's not easy to impress me, and it's hard to teach me anything I can't learn on my own. But one person teaches me every day and challenges me in ways I never dreamed imaginable, and that's my beautiful and bright daughter, Pilar. She's my living proof that emotions make you weak, because when it comes to her, I'm just a daddy in love with his little girl. She's smart and beautiful like her mother, and she's my reason for coming back from the dark side of intensity and competition and unyielding pressure, into the light and love she melts me with every day of my life. My deepest wish is that everything I do makes her as proud of me as I am of her.

I'm telling you that because my advice to my daughter is the same advice I pass along to you, so you know it's the truth:

Every dream you imagine, everything you see and hear and feel in your sleep, that's not a fantasy, that's your deep instinct telling you it can all be real. Follow those visions and dreams and desires, and believe what you know. Only you can turn those dreams into reality. Never stop until you do.

The greatest battles you will ever fight are with yourself, and you must always be your toughest opponent.

Always demand more of yourself than others demand of you. Be honest with yourself, and you'll be able to meet every challenge with confidence and the deep belief that you are prepared for anything. Life can be complicated; the truth is not.

I truly believe I have zero limitations. You should believe the same about yourself. Listen to your instincts. They're telling you the truth.

I want the satisfaction of knowing that every move I make, every thought, every idea, every action takes me further than anyone else has ever gone and makes me better at what I do than anyone else in the world. That's what drives me. Whatever drives you, let it take you where you want to be. Everything you want can be yours. Be a Cleaner and go get it.

Be relentless.

Done.

Next.

ACKNOWLEDGMENTS

Special thanks to everyone who made this book possible, especially Scribner Senior Editor Shannon Welch and my relentless agent and coauthor, Shari Wenk, who prove that women are truly the ultimate Cleaners.

Also thanks to the rest of the Cleaners at Scribner, particularly Susan Moldow, Nan Graham, and John Glynn, and to all the athletes who have trusted me with their talents over the years, and believe as I do that there is no such thing as being good enough.

Read on for an excerpt from

Tim Grover's Jump Attack

Coming soon from Scribner

Near the end of Michael Jordan's career with the Bulls, he agreed to allow a camera crew to follow him around for a documentary on his last season in Chicago. Early one morning—maybe 6:00 a.m., it was dark outside and Michael's kids were still asleep—the crew came to his house for a rare glimpse into his private gym where we trained. The video has never been released, but I can tell you how it began:

The cameraman noticed a poster on the wall, a classic shot of MJ soaring through the air with the caption, HOW DOES MICHAEL FLY? He zoomed in on the poster, then turned the camera to Michael and asked him, "How *do* you fly?"

Michael just laughed, shook his head, pointed across the gym at me, and said, "Ask him."

Good question.

No doubt Michael's genetics gave him a physical advantage: he has huge hands, long limbs, and predominately fast-twitch muscles. But contrary to popular legend, he is not a freak of nature. I know people mean it as a compliment when they say that about him, but I think of it as an insult, because it suggests he didn't have to work for his success. In fact, there are plenty of athletes who share his physical abilities, and in some cases even exceed them. But he has mental toughness that exceeds anyone else's physical toughness, and that's ultimately what separates merely great athletes from iconic superstars. That's why Kobe Bryant, in his thirties, can outplay guys who are much younger. Like Michael, he has the mentality and focus and relentless drive to maximize his skills, push beyond, and never stop working to improve.

So there are undoubtedly many factors that allowed Michael to fly. But when he pointed at me in his gym that morning, this is what he meant: we trained in a way that maximized his abilities and gifts, so he could reach his ultimate potential in every way. And that training—the "secret" to Michael's explosiveness and the power he had to launch himself through the air—is the basis for my program, *Jump Attack*.

Jump Attack is a total-body workout—legs, arms, core—that delivers results, whether you're a young player getting started or an experienced athlete looking to improve . . . and we all have room to improve.

It's not easy. But if you want proof that *Jump Attack* works, just ask any of my clients. It's the same program I've used with the pros since I first developed it with Michael in the 1990s.

Increasing vertical jump and explosiveness is one of the most difficult things to accomplish in athletic training; it requires specific muscles to be activated and firing simultaneously for a prolonged period of time. If you're doing it correctly, everything works together for extraordinary results; the right training will send you soaring over the competition. The wrong training will leave you flat on your feet.

Give me twelve weeks and your best effort, and I'll give you a complete plan that delivers:

- Explosive athleticism for ultimate performance in all sports and activities
- Increased muscle mass, power, speed, and agility
- A tighter, leaner physique
- Mental toughness and endurance
- Effective rest and recovery
- Optimal nutrition
- Injury prevention

The key to the program is my Explosive Sequences, the critical component for developing the body and skills of a winner. For twelve weeks, you'll use ten unique all-new workouts to master the sequences, consistently increasing your vertical jump, overall athleticism, and muscle mass with each phase of the program.

Here's a look at the *Jump Attack* system:

Weeks 1–3: Phase One—Don't Think

If you're thinking, you're failing. We're preparing your body, your ligaments, your muscles, your mind, testing you mentally so you can be ready to get through the next phases.

These are simple but challenging isometric workouts—no weights—that make you sweat like crazy and ignite your muscles to react as never before. Don't think about what you're doing, just focus on the results and get it done.

Day 1: Endurance Legs #1
Day 2: Endurance Total Body #1
Day 3: Stretch and Recover
Day 4: Endurance Legs #2
Day 5: Endurance Total Body #2
Day 6: Stretch and Recover
Day 7: Rest

Week 4: Rest, Test, and Recovery

After each phase, you'll take a week to rest your body and recover from the intense work you've been doing. You'll test yourself twice during each recovery week to measure your progress. Don't be discouraged if you don't see quick results; the payoff comes at the end of the entire program.

Weeks 5–7: Phase Two—Attack

Now your body is ready for the hard work; get ready to to push yourself harder than you ever have. We're adding weights, overloading the muscles, getting them ready to apply more force into the ground, and teaching them to fire over and over, without fatigue or weakness.

Day 1: Power Legs
Day 2: Power Body
Day 3: Stretch and Recover
Day 4: Power Legs
Day 5: Power Body
Day 6: Stretch and Recover
Day 7: Rest

Week 8: Rest, Test, and Recovery

Another week to rest and recover. Stay active; use each recovery week to play your sport, and let your body start learning how to use your new abilities and skills.

Weeks 9–11: Phase Three—Relentless

Anyone can start something; it takes a winner to finish. If you're still working to get results, you are truly relentless—a lot of pros don't make it this far. Phase Three combines all the workouts from the first two phases and kicks everything into high gear. Stay with it a little longer and accomplish what you started.

Day 1: Explosive Legs
Day 2: Explosive Body
Day 3: Stretch and Recover
Day 4: Explosive Legs
Day 5: Explosive Body

Day 6: Stretch and Recover
Day 7: Rest

Week 12: Rest and Testing

Congratulations, you've completed the *Jump Attack* program. But you still need the final week to rest your muscles and let your body fully recover. Take your final two tests, record your results, and get ready to take your game to a whole new level.

• • •

Jump Attack is more than just a workout; it's a complete program that addresses all your athletic needs and issues.

Train the Mind to Train the Body

Fact: You can't be physically tough until you're mentally tough. . . . You must be unbeatable from the neck up before you can be unbeatable from the neck down. Based on the principles of *Relentless,* I'll show you how to get comfortable being uncomfortable and prepare your mind and body to reach a whole new level of success.

Getting Started

We'll test your vertical jump for the first time (you'll repeat the test several times throughout the program) and record your starting stats so you can measure your progress. Learn the rules of perfect form and go through the *Jump Attack* warm-up for flexibility and injury prevention.

Jump Attack Fuel

You don't put cheap gasoline into an elite automobile, and you don't fuel an athletic body with junk food. I'll share the nutrition plan I give my players, including a complete list of dos and don'ts, as well as advice on supplements and other performance enhancers.

Injury Prevention, Rest, and Recovery

No matter how great the athlete, injuries happen. We'll talk about preventing them before they occur and recovering safely when they do. As I tell my players after an injury: I don't want you to come back as good as you were before; I want you to come back stronger than ever.

Jump Attack Maintenance

Being the best means never being satisfied; you never stop working and improving. That's how the best get better. No matter how good you are, you can always do more. At the end of the twelve weeks, the maintenance phase gives you the tools you need to build on the gains you've made and set your sights on a whole new level of excellence.

The Workout Journal

A training log is your most important workout partner; you can't measure success at the end if you don't know where you began. The book includes blank pages for recording results and keeping a record of weights/reps/stats.

Attack Athletics Q&A

All your training questions answered, including a few you didn't think to ask.

• • •

This is the blueprint for jumping higher, moving quicker, packing on muscle, and developing explosive power. Your job is to follow the plan and work hard. That's it. It takes no talent to work hard; anyone can do it. The greats might be born with extraordinary talent, but they know the truth: it's not enough to get to the top; and you have to fight to stay there.

If you're serious about that fight, if you're ready to change your body and your game, if you're committed to showing up and doing the work, you're on a journey that will set you apart from the competition and take you places you never imagined. *Jump Attack* takes the mental fitness you mastered in *Relentless* and completes the mind-body connection. *Relentless* made you mentally tough; now you're ready to be physically tough.

It works.

During the 2012 NBA finals, I spent five days in Miami with my longtime client Dwyane Wade, trying to get the most out of a damaged knee that would need surgery after the season. The work we did—sometimes at 2:00 a.m.—will remain private, but at the end of the finals, as the Heat were crowned the NBA champs and the champagne flowed in the locker room, Miami GM and NBA legend Pat Riley came up to me and said, "I'd love to know how you got Dwyane so explosive in just a few days."

The answer is the premise for *Jump Attack.*

You'll need more than the five days I spent with Dwyane in Miami, but the work I did with him—and what I do with all my players—is the basis for what I'm giving you in this program. For more than two decades I've watched and trained the best of the best; I study how they improve, what works and what doesn't. In my business, success is in the details: if your leg twitches, if your shot is off, if you're fatiguing faster or slower than you did before, I'm going to notice. I'm putting everything I've learned, everything I've taught, everything I know into *Jump Attack*. This is how the best get better, and you can too.

● ● ●

For more information on *Jump Attack* and Tim Grover, visit www.attackathletics.com.